Beyond Nakedness

Beyond Nakedness

by
Paul Ableman

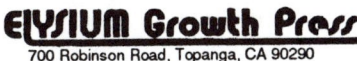

ELYSIUM Growth Press
700 Robinson Road, Topanga, CA 90290

BEYOND NAKEDNESS
Published by Elysium Growth Press
in the United States of America
American edition © 1985
Second Edition © 1993

First published in Great Brirain by
Orbis Publishing Limited, London, 1982
© 1982 by Paul Ableman

Printed in the United States of America
ISBN: 0-910550-56-5

CONTENTS

THE HAIRLESS APE

There are still a few naked tribes left in the world. Whether they are truly naked will be discussed later in this book, but for the present purpose, certain peoples in South America, in New Guinea and in Africa can be considered naked. We mean by this that such ornaments, tattoos or deliberate scars as they display on their bodies do not have the function of genital concealment.

The aim of this book is to examine what nakedness means to different peoples, and particularly what it has meant throughout the 'civilized ages' when concealment, more or less thorough, has been customary.

Man without clothes appears to be a peculiarly, perhaps uniquely, naked animal. Desmond Morris called his witty and informative account of our species, as seen from the perspective of a zoologist, *The Naked Ape*. There is, however, a false implication in this title, which is that other apes are clothed. The true antithesis of the naked body is not the hairy but the clothed body. But it is clear what Morris meant. Man's hairlessness seems to give him a peculiarly blatant nakedness as compared to our furred and hairy fellow mammals. His ostentatious display of skin, a membrane which is both the container of the body's functional components and the boundary between the self and the world, is supplemented by his upright posture. Man appears to be flaunting all his biological mysteries, which, in most other species, are shrouded in hair and rendered to some extent inconspicuous by posture. Looking at a naked human being from the front, we see the navel, which once connected him or her with the mother, the genitals, which will produce the next generation, the breasts of the female or vestigial nipples of the male, the panel of assorted sensory equipment on the face, the excretory apparatus pitched in what some poets have found to be distressing proximity to the reproductive organs, and many details of muscular and skeletal structure. In reality no more naked than a baboon, man seems to be utterly bare.

Another class of warm-blooded creatures which shares this surface nakedness is the group of aquatic mammals. Dolphins and whales, like man, have a smooth hairless surface. In their case, the smooth finish is designed to facilitate motion through the water. But in colour, in general concealment of reproductive organs, and because water provides a veil, the aquatic mammals do not seem anything like as naked as we are.

Man is, in fact, a biological oddity. This remark may be challenged by some members of our intensely narcissistic species. Although civilized people are, and always have been, diffident about exposing their naked bodies, there is no lack of evidence that we have a high regard for our hairless forms. We have filled our public places with representations, often naked, of our bodies. Stylized and idealized, but naked, figure paintings grace our most elegant interiors. Metaphysical philosophers have endeavoured to derive absolute laws of proportion, and even keys to space and time, from segments of the human body. Horse-lovers and dog-lovers enthuse about the lines of these 'noble' beasts, and those of larger sympathies are capable of finding beauty in most of the forms of nature, but there is no doubt that, generally, we regard ourselves as being several cuts above the rest of creation in terms of aesthetic excellence. There are, nevertheless, valid grounds for regarding ourselves as oddities.

How did we get to be upright hairless apes?

The truth is, no one really knows and the range, and bizarre ingenuity, of some of the theories testify to how obscure the matter remains.

Adult human beings have a lot in common with unborn apes. This has led to the proposition that *homo sapiens* really represents not an evolutionary advance from a primitive primate ancestor but a kind of fixation (with later development) of a primitive ape fetus. This unlikely process is not unknown elsewhere in nature. It is called neoteny. There is a famous example in the axolotl, a kind of salamander that, according to conditions, either grows to adult form or remains a tadpole all its life. In the latter case, the 'ripe' tadpole can reproduce like an adult. There are some rather striking confirmations of the fixation theory. The most surprising is the fact that fetal female apes – those still in the womb – possess hymens while young and adult apes do not. The hymen is the tough, elastic membrane which seals the entrance to the vagina in human beings. If we were more 'advanced' than apes, proponents of this theory say, we should also have lost our hymens but, of course, the human female has this membrane. Human beings also present several other fetal ape characteristics. Like the intrauterine apes, we are relatively hairless. We have the same body/head-size ratio. There are, however, also differences. Some people have suggested that, as a species, we are the result of 'differential infantilism', deriving some of our characteristics from fetal apes and some from other sources. However, even if our hairlessness were originally a product of neoteny, it would still be unclear why we have remained naked when virtually every other mammal has, over the millennia, clothed itself in an insulating coat of hair.

Let us look briefly at some of the other theories which account for our hairlessness. Perhaps the most picturesque is the 'aquatic theory'. This states that when our primate forebears left the forests and took to an upright life on the plains, they found getting enough to eat very difficult. They were outpaced by almost every other sizeable creature about, which made both obtaining food, and avoiding becoming food, extremely trying. Seeking a secure food supply they eventually found one in the shellfish on the sea-shore. The quest for such nutriment led man into deeper and deeper waters until at last he became virtually an aquatic mammal. The chief objective confirmation of this theory is that the hairs on our backs (for we are not, of course, really a 'hairless' species but a finely-haired species) are disposed in a way that would minimize water resistance, and which contrasts with the hair lines on other primates. There is also the matter of subcutaneous fat. In common with seals, whales and dolphins, man has quite a thick layer of fat beneath his skin. Indeed, it is his chief protection in the naked state. No other primate has this. The chief objection to the aquatic theory is that it is purely speculative. In refutation, it might be argued that if we were doing so well in the sea why did we not go on to join the, generally speaking, highly successful aquatic mammals and reside there permanently or, like the seals, semi-permanently? Why did we return, with the same miserable disadvantages as before, to an unequal struggle on land?

Our hairlessness has been seen as an attempt to minimize insect parasitism, as a form of sexual signalling, as a way of keeping cool in the hot plains – and other hypotheses as well have been proposed to account for it. All these hypotheses suffer from the same defect. They would, or could, apply to other species too, especially to plains foragers like the baboon. But man is the only ape that has shed his hair, expanded his brain and developed arched feet and superb grasping hands. And no one really knows why, or has even produced a satisfactory working theory regarding the matter.

It is, however, worth recalling that a similar development occurred to another of the more intelligent mammals. Our cave-dwelling ancestors before the last ice age left pictures of the animals they hunted on the walls of their caverns. Among these was the mammoth, forebear of the modern elephant. The mammoth was covered in a thick coat of hair. We know this because several have been found preserved intact in permafrost. We have not been lucky enough to find any mammoth-hunters similarly preserved but perhaps if we did we would discover that man has not always been a hairless or naked ape. The artist-hunters who had brains the same size as ours, might have been as thickly coated as the mammoths they hunted. There is no way of knowing since hair rots away. If mammoths were known, as our ancestors are known, exclusively from their skeletal remains, we might be disposed to regard hairlessness as just as much a quality of the *proboscidea* (elephants) as it is of *homo sapiens*, and if the mammoths lost their hair so might our ancestors have done. In other words, we may well have become, in essentials, fully human before we became hairless. In truth, a large brain is the most striking physiological characteristic of *homo sapiens* and even that characteristic is shared by dolphins and elephants. What really makes us different from all other creatures is our culture. So perhaps it would be most appropriate to think of ourselves as 'cultured apes'.

ADAM AND EVE

In countries having a Christian tradition, two chief explanations are offered for the presence of human beings on the earth. One is natural and the other supernatural. The first is, of course, Darwin's theory of evolution by natural selection which, 120 years after having been first propounded, survives relatively intact and is accepted, with some modifications, by most thinking people. It remains the orthodox explanation for the multiplicity of species on the earth and for the rise of increasingly complex forms leading to man. Such speculative opposition as it meets in the scientific community is largely concerned with detail.

For one and a half thousand million years, single-celled organisms, the blue-green bacteria, were the sole inhabitants of the earth. This means that these microscopic beings have been around longer than any other life form. Simplicity can usually be equated with durability. All present-day living things are descended from these micro-organisms and it is a nice question as to whether the gulf which separates a blue-green bacterium from a man is greater than that which separates it from a grain of sand. The second half of life's 3,000 million year presence on this planet saw the relatively rapid evolution of all kinds of plant and animal life which now exist and of the many forms which have become extinct. As evolution advanced, its pace increased. From blue-green bacteria to sponges took 2,000 million years. From tree-shrews to man took a mere three million. In other words, mind started exploding on the planet. That, in brief outline, is the scientific account of our origins.

The alternative theological explanation for the presence of man is, of course, the one contained in the *Book of Genesis*. According to this, God created the world in seven days and stocked it with immutable forms. Then he created man in his own image and woman from a rib of man. These primal human beings were called Adam and Eve.

Almost all human cultures produce 'creation myths' of one kind or another. Often a god or spirit is seen as the primal artificer. Sometimes life emerges from a kind of creative cloud or from a biological constituent, like a drop of blood. The need to explain our origins, and indeed universal origins, is a powerful one. But the Judaeo-Christian myth has been exceptionally influential. Darwin himself was a Christian, and Christianity is so thoroughly intricated into the culture of the West, including its scientific culture, that men who can recognize the creation myths of simpler people as literary creations may still accept the literal truth of *Genesis*. Indeed, what might be called naive belief is undergoing a revival, and very sophisticated writers are attacking Darwinism and defending *Genesis*. The psychological dilemma of people raised in both a scientific and a Christian tradition has perhaps never been more poignantly expressed than in Edmund Gosse's fine and moving book *Father and Son*. Edmund's father, Philip Gosse, was both a Christian of the most fundamentalist kind, one of the Plymouth Brethren, and a scrupulous biologist who was himself responsible, at the time of Darwin, for discoveries that tended to confirm evolution and discredit *Genesis*. His mental sufferings were pitiable and ultimately he was driven to renounce science. Some modern scientists still experience the same sense of division between the message of the natural world and that of the supernatural. But most scientists who are also Christians would now resolve the problem by accepting Darwinism as structurally accurate and the account in *Genesis* as being poetic or mythical truth.

Nothing in the *Genesis* account is more haunting, or more durably relevant to human culture, than the story of Adam and Eve. It is, of course, well known but in order to look at some of its implications, here is a brief recapitulation.

God provides a garden for Adam and Eve. The garden is stocked with 'every tree that is pleasing to the sight and good for food'. Adam and Eve live there naked and are completely content, or almost completely content. They would be totally satisfied with their lot were it not for one thing. There is a single tree in the garden which they have been forbidden by God to touch, the tree of the knowledge of Good and Evil. One day, the serpent, at this stage apparently an upright (in the postural sense) creature, tempts Eve. He tells her that if she eats the fruit of this tree, she and Adam will acquire god-like powers. The two human beings eat. And the first consequence of their action is that they realize that they are *naked*. Shame envelops them. They 'sewed fig leaves together and made themselves aprons'. God learns of their disobedience. They are banished from the Garden and punished, the woman with increased pain in childbearing (a little oddly since she has as yet borne no children), and the man by henceforth having to toil for his bread. The serpent is condemned to crawl on his belly and is cursed with the eternal enmity of Eve.

The awesome power of this myth stems from the fact that it puts in a highly compressed, poetically exact form a central truth about life on earth which in no way conflicts with Darwinism. This is the change from an animal to a human state. We may classify this variously as the change from unselfconsciousness to self-consciousness; the change from timelessness to the awareness of time; the change from unthinking participation in the natural world to conceptual separation from it.

The awareness of time which characterizes the human state means the constant awareness of death, and this is the most terrible product of the change from an animal to a human condition. Death, as it is known to man, has no counterpart in nature. Man's awareness of death means that he necessarily sees himself as participating in natural process. But this objectification is, ironically, also the cause of man's sense of detachment or alienation from natural processes, which has in the long term led to our scientific-technical culture.

Nevertheless the immediate consequence of the expulsion from the Garden of Eden – or from the unselfconscious, natural state – according to the *Genesis* account, is a realization of nakedness.

What does this biblical nakedness symbolize? Adam and Eve in the Garden are not good. Nor are they evil. They exist, like animals, in an amoral state that precedes the generation of good or evil, that is, of morality. Now, of course, animals have no morality. A tiger throttling an antelope is not committing murder. A baboon mounting its daughter is not guilty of either rape or incest. Without a knowledge of good and evil, and the laws that flow from this knowledge, moral qualities cannot exist. Adam and Eve discover them first in the awareness of their own nakedness. The clear implication in *Genesis* is that Adam and Eve's new-found knowledge of good and evil had directed their attention not to the nakedness of their bodies in general, but to the nakedness of their genitals. They do not make themselves cloaks or suits or dresses but *aprons*. Good and evil are perceived as being associated with sexuality and reproduction and the reproductive parts instantly become shameful, base, evil and dangerous. Henceforth they have to be concealed. Thus, the anonymous genius who set down the Garden of Eden story located sexuality at the core of human morality. Three thousand years later, Sigmund Freud did the same. The nakedness of Adam and Eve symbolizes the original innocence of non-human nature and the aprons symbolize the later ambiguous labyrinth of human morality and civilization.

One further point is relevant here. The serpent, when it tempts Eve, appears to be, like the other beasts, basically equal to the human inhabitants of the Garden. After Adam and Eve's discovery of good and evil, which initiates a moral view of the universe, the serpent is reduced to ground level. This seems to represent metaphorically what has actually happened in the world. With increasing self-conscious-ness, man has separated himself more and more from all other living things until now he holds absolute power over them. We can do what we like with beasts and plants and we are so powerful that we could exterminate them all and ourselves as well. Paradoxically, this human scientific advance, by making it seem that man is somehow categori-cally different even from other primates, never mind, say, jellyfish, has made it easier for a kind of highly sophisticated, classically educated intellectual to argue *against* the scientific account of evolution and *for* the literal truth of the Old Testament myth. We have so outstripped the other inhabitants of the Garden – that some of us find it hard to believe that we are related.

Adam and Eve were originally naked. Animals are naked. A few contemporary tribes are still naked. Are nakedness and innocence linked? Is naked man essentially pre-cultural man and does conceal-ment of the body indicate developing cultural complexity? In a very broad sense, the answer to these questions is undoubtedly 'yes'. True, there have been very simple and primitive cultures which, for one reason or another, have been heavily clothed. The Eskimos are an obvious example. Although the connection between climatic con-ditions and degree of bodily covering is by no means a simple one, 'hairless apes' could not survive in the Arctic except in borrowed skins. Some cultures, such as the Japanese, in which nakedness, if not the rule, was at least quite common, have been complex. Nevertheless, there is a broad correspondence between bodily concealment and the degree of what is traditionally called civilization. The transition from big-brained primates to *homo sapiens* is also a transition from nakedness to clothes. And as soon as man is clothed he bears a visual sign of his separateness and uniqueness. It is interesting that the Eskimos who are clothed by necessity but who nevertheless live very intimately with nature strip naked inside their igloos without any self-consciousness or shame.

Now true nakedness is rare. By true nakedness is meant, in this context, the nakedness of people whose body surface is both un-adorned (with clothing or ornamentation) and unmodified (by tattoo-ing, painting or scarification). But, for the present, 'nakedness' can be taken as meaning unconcealed. Thus a naked tribe is one in which, although ornaments or even clothing may be worn, no systematic attempt is made to hide the body or its functions.

Generally speaking, people who live on familiar terms with their own bodies also live on easy terms with their environment. Co-operation with nature, rather than an attempt to dominate it, is characteristic of their life-style. An extreme example of this came to light eight years ago when a completely unknown tribe, the Tasaday, was discovered in the jungle of the Phillipines. This gentle people was at a very primitive stage of cultural development. It had language but practically no other attributes of civilization. The Tasaday lived naked and their only shelter was caves. The interesting, and indeed astonish-ing, fact about their life-style was that they made no attempt whatsoever to modify their environment. They lived by gathering and they shared their caves with any other life-forms that cared to occupy them. Since these included venomous snakes, the forbearance of the Tasaday was remarkable. Obviously, like Adam and Eve in Eden, they made no distinction between themselves and any other living beings. It never occurred to them to modify the scheme of things for their own benefit or convenience.

This is an extreme example. But in New Guinea and the Brazilian jungle live a number of tribes that have evolved simple cultures which are static and in fine ecological balance with their surroundings. They build shelters, even large and imposing ones, and they have hunting weapons and simple food-preparing equipment, but little or no agriculture. Their societies are integrated into the natural scheme.

Margaret Mead, in her study of the Arapesh peoples of the Sepik River in New Guinea, writes:

> Neither little girls nor little boys wear any clothes until they are
> four or five; they are taught to accept their physiological differ-

ences without any shame or embarrassment ... Thus there develops in the children an easy, happy-go-lucky familiarity with the bodies of both sexes, a familiarity uncomplicated by shame, coupled with a premium upon warm, all-over physical contact.

It would be agreeable to be able to state that life in the real Edens of the world is always simple, uncomplicated, affectionate and wholesome. There are indeed examples of such idyllic societies. But nakedness alone is not enough to ensure blissful innocence and the temperamental and cultural disparities among naked peoples are, if anything, more pronounced than those among 'civilized' peoples. In the Brazilian jungles tribes of happy, healthy Indians live alongside tribes of savage drug addicts. In New Guinea, the gentle Arapesh have as neighbours the ferocious Mundugamor, head-hunters and cannibals. Margaret Mead was warned by Arapesh elders: 'You are going up the Sepik River, where the people are very fierce, where they eat men ... Do not be misled by your experiences among us. We are another kind.'

But one thing is common to virtually all naked peoples: an intense interest in the human body and its functions, including its sexual functions. Cultural activity revolves around the body. Dance is the characteristic art form, and magic, which is common in nearly all primitive cultures, is concerned largely with the body and its products.

Children in naked cultures do not grow up in ignorance of sex. They have opportunities to observe adults making love and are rarely restrained from sexual experimentation themselves. The following passage from *Cult of the Sacred Spear* by Brian Hugh Macdermot, an account of life with the totally naked Nuer tribe of Ethiopia, describes an attitude to infantile sexual exploration which is common among naked peoples:

> Children ... enjoy a freedom in their games which might shock the modern world. One day, I saw a boy and girl aged about 7 or 8 disappear into the grass where they attempted to make love. The elders asked: what harm can they do? No babies will result.

Likewise, masturbation and almost all forms of erotic play and experimentation are regarded with amused tolerance. Obviously, growing up in a naked society means that basic physiological processes are seen and understood. Birth, copulation and suckling are all witnessed and discussed. But there is one physiological phenomenon which almost always perplexes primitives. This is menstruation. Lacking sophisticated medical knowledge, they find its reason obscure and they usually resort to mythological explanations, often related to the moon, as Penelope Shuttle and Peter Redgrove show in their richly metaphorical treatise, *The Wise Wound*. The periodicity of the menstrual cycle, which is roughly similar to the lunar cycle, although only haphazardly in phase with it, suggests the connection. The Maori see menstruation as a sickness caused by the moon, and the Papuans believe that the moon has intercourse with girls and causes them to bleed.

For many cultures, a girl's first menstruation symbolizes the transition from childhood to womanhood, and thus becomes the occasion for an initiation ceremony.

H. Crawford Angus (quoted in Havelock Ellis's *Psychology of Sex*) describes the Azimba girls of Central Africa:

> At the first sign of menstruation the girl is taken by her mother out of the village to a grass hut prepared for her where only the women are allowed to visit her. At the end of menstruation, she is taken to a secluded spot and the women dance round her, no men being present.

Amongst the Thlinkeet Eskimo women, the puberty rites were far more stringent. 'At puberty they were secluded, sometimes for a whole year, being kept in darkness, suffering and filth.' To this oppressive régime was attributed the 'modest reserve and meditation' for which these women were famous.

Primitives may not understand the true nature of menstruation, but they do perceive its connection with female sexuality in general, and they are certainly not ignorant of its occurrence. In the West, improved sex education probably means that nowadays most children acquire at least a hazy technical understanding of the phenomenon. But until quite recently, it was possible for a man to reach maturity in total ignorance of this important fact about female life. Alfred Hitchcock recalled how, in his early days as a film director, he presented himself on a beach to direct an aquatic scene. In those technically unsophisticated times, this meant that just he, the cameraman and the actress needed to be present. After Hitchcock and the cameraman had waited for some time, a messenger arrived with the information that the actress could not go into the water that day.

'Why not?' asked Hitchcock.

'You understand – she cannot go in the water today.'

Hitchcock did not understand and, under the impression that his star was crazy, abandoned shooting for that morning. It is perhaps a poignant reflection that a modern man, wielding the (then) most advanced technological equipment, had contrived to reach maturity in utter ignorance of a fact, and a mystery, familiar to every child in a primitive society.

Another physiological fact which is viewed very differently by primitive and civilized societies is excretion. Margaret Mead, again writing about the Arapesh, states that 'Excretion is not a matter about which privacy is insisted upon for small children. Indeed adults merely go casually to the edge of the village. Their attitude is characterized by shyness rathan than shame.'

Naked people are not equipped with special sanitary equipment. Since their 'dirt' is not whisked away through underground pipes as it is for us, they incorporate the process of excretion into their world view simply and naturally. But they do usually have a sense of cleanliness. This contrasts strongly with the anthropoid apes. According to Desmond Morris, '99% of abandoned gorilla nests . . . had gorilla dung inside them and in 73% the animals had actually been lying in it.'

Nakedness, or near-nakedness, is not incompatible with modesty. According to Yolanda and Robert Murphy in *Women of the Forest*, among the Mundurucu Indians of Brazil the women wear nothing and the men just a bark cloth belt and a palm-leaf penis-sheath. Nevertheless, they display a great sense of personal modesty. The women always sit on the ground with their legs stretched out in front of them and close together. They are quite happy to show the breasts and pubic hair but not the genitals. Men take great care to conceal their penises. When bathing, the men turn their backs on their fellows, remove the penis sheath and slip quickly into the water, staying submerged until they are ready to come out, when they replace the sheath as quickly as possible. Likewise, little girls in some naked African tribes are taught how to sit in such a way as to conceal their vulvas.

This modesty is less likely, especially in the case of women, to derive from shame than from belief in magic. Since menstruation is a great and potent mystery, the female genitals are thought to have great magical powers which are usually considered, at least by males, to be powers for evil. The Kiwai Papuans consider that all magic is directly or indirectly derived from the female genitals, which they believe to be as perilous as 'an open grave', an image that Freudians will appreciate. In this culture, the men are naked but the women cover the lower part of their bodies, because of the dread power of their genitals.

John Langdon-Davies, author of *The Future of Nakedness* wrote as recently as 1929:

> The present of nakedness can be stated in a brief sentence: nakedness today is a crime in all civilized countries and a sin in all Christian congregations; it is an unnatural and vicious condition of the human body; it is the fruit of that forbidden tree the eating of which men have no intention of risking again.

He is perhaps overstating the case somewhat for the time at which he was writing, when nudist colonies thrived in Germany and existed in England and elsewhere; and his conclusion would need considerably modifying if applied to the present day, when charter companies fly large numbers of people to the French Riviera and Yugoslavia for 'naturist' holidays. It is certainly true, however, that in our culture public nakedness remains unlawful. The body must be hidden. It is still possible, perhaps common, to grow up 'in all civilized countries' with only a vague knowledge of the human body and its functions.

This alienation from the body is reflected in literature. Again, some qualification must be made as regards modern, particularly post-war, literature but one could still spend hours in a modern library, taking down book after book at random, and find little evidence that human beings have bodies and practically none as to what those bodies are really like. *Everything else*, from the distant reaches of the cosmos to all the activities, including war, that take place on this planet, is abundantly documented. But for two and a half thousand years literature other than medical literature has either ignored the body and its functions or consigned it to the underworld of smut, pornography and the 'dirty' joke.

The situation is very different with primitives. Of course, they generally have no written literature but they always produce a wealth of orally transmitted myth and song, sometimes, indeed, long epic works. In these, an important subject is the body and its functions. Sexuality pervades primitive myth.

It is as if, by donning 'aprons', Adam and Eve sealed off their bodies and forced man's thought outwards towards all the rest of creation. Freud called this process 'repression' and maintained that it was essential for the growth of civilization. This is not the place to discuss whether the price has been too high or whether, indeed, such exile from our bodies was really necessary to build complex societies. But it is the right place to note the fact that we civilized peoples always have been, and basically still are, distanced from our own bodies.

From the sixteenth century onwards, clothed Europeans regularly encountered naked primitives all over the world. The Spanish in South America came upon naked Indians in Brazil and elsewhere. Captain Cook found naked, or unconcealed, islanders in Polynesia and New Zealand. Later British, French, Germans and Portuguese, among others, came into contact with naked Africans. The results of these meetings were usually lamentable for the simpler cultures. The Europeans exploited them economically and sexually. Sometimes, indeed, they exterminated them. But it was not until the eighteenth and, especially, the nineteenth centuries that they made much attempt to change them. Then came the missionaries, and the first aspect of primitive life to experience their reforming zeal was inevitably the nakedness of the potential new recruits to Christianity. Doubtless most of the missionaries meant well, but they proved a greater force for ruin than the simpler and more brutal traders and explorers.

The missionaries were usually disconcerted to find that the biblically recommended act of 'clothing the naked', far from producing an improvement in native morals, almost always resulted in a deterioration. What the missionaries were inadvertently doing was recreating the Garden of Eden situation. Naked, the primitive cultures had shown no prurient concern with the body, although morals were often, by civilized standards, rather lax. Indeed, some primitives never connected copulation with pregnancy and childbirth, since all women copulated freely from puberty but not all women conceived. Most simple cultures, however, were not as promiscuous as this and there was almost always some morality, usually connected with taboo and kinship groups. Then again, what Desmond Morris calls 'pairbonding', and we call marriage, was common, and some restrictions on free sexuality were usually imposed on married people. In some primitive communities, indeed, the penalty for adultery could be of biblical ferocity. Nonetheless, the morality was normally geared to the naked state of the culture. The missionaries, with their cotton shorts and dresses, disrupted this. Naked people actually feel shame when they are first dressed. They develop an exaggerated awareness of the body. It is as if Adam and Eve's 'aprons' *generated* the 'knowledge of good and evil' rather than being its consequence. But the disruption caused by the missionaries went far deeper as a result of the vital fact that very few primitives are totally naked. They almost all have ornamentation or body-modification of some kind, *which plays a central role in their culture.*

The aborigines of Australia are one of the simplest and barest of cultures, yet they are not naked, according to A.P. Elkin.

> A pubic tassel made of fur string is worn, though it is not an
> effective covering. Indeed, in the case of the men, this tassel or the
> pearl-shell pubic pendant is really a sign of having reached a
> prescribed stage in initiation. It corresponds to the 'lodge apron'.
> Girls who wear these fur tassels have reached the age of marriage.

Into this simple but successful culture comes the missionary, and obliterates the key signs beneath his cheap Western clothing. Among many primitives, tattooing, scarification and ornamentation convey highly elaborate information which may, in fact, be the central regulatory force in the society. The missionary thus, at one blow, annihilates a culture. It was probably no less traumatic for a primitive society to be suddenly clothed than it would be for our's to be suddenly stripped naked.

And if primitives lost their culture, they also lost their environment. They lost the sun, the rain, the grass underfoot, the foliage which brushed their skin as they moved through forest or jungle, the water of lake, river or sea slipping past their bodies, above all the ceaseless communion with the wind. Anyone who has ever spent any time naked outdoors knows that the play of the elements over the body produces an ever-changing response that may reach almost erotic intensity. The skin becomes alive and responsive and a whole new spectrum of sensation is generated. Clothe the body and this rich communion is replaced by mere fortuitous, and often irritating, contact with inert fabric. It is a huge impoverishment and its measure can perhaps best be judged by the reluctance of the Indians of Tierra del Fuego, who live in a climate so harsh that Darwin observed snow melting on the naked breasts of women, to adopt protective clothing. They preferred dermal contact with the environment, hostile though it was, to the loss of sensation implied by wearing clothes.

A classic encounter between Western civilization and Eden took place with the arrival of Europeans in Polynesia. Perhaps the foremost authority on the subject, or at least on its erotic dimension, is Bengt Danielsson, the anthropologist, who lived for many yers in the islands. *Love in the South Seas* is his account of what he found there.

> Since the first island within the huge Polynesian triangle delimited
> by Hawaii, New Zealand and Easter Island was discovered in 1595
> by the Spaniard Mendana ... the Polynesians have enjoyed an
> unrivalled reputation for their sexual freedom and hospitality.

Chapter after chapter documents the superb aesthetic voluptuousness of these islanders. It should perhaps be stated at the outset that the Polynesians, generally speaking, were not a naked people. But they were an unconcealed one. There was modesty but no mystery about the body and its functions. Children under five went naked. Nakedness above the waist was normal and total nakedness, as well as public sexual acitivity, was common on various occasions. The old Polynesians, a most fastidious people, bathed twice daily and perfumed their skins. When a woman was in labour (and childbirth for them was, and remains, for reasons that are still mysterious, much easier than it is for women in most other parts of the world), crowds would collect to watch and applaud the delivery. Erotic games were not only tolerated but encouraged, although only within a given age group. Adults of opposite sex meeting in the bush would usually make love. Mothers encouraged their children to masturbate. Polygamy was common.

And yet this society was not anarchic. There were definite rules which governed behaviour, including sexual behaviour, but they were geared to maximizing, rather than minimizing, sensual satisfaction.

The naturalist Commerson, who sailed with the French navigator Bougainville, wrote in 1769 that the Tahitians 'know no other god than love. Every day is consecrated to him. The whole island is his temple in which all the women are idols and all the men worshippers. And what women!' In fact, the Tahitians, a stone-age people who nevertheless generated a culture of great elegance, did know other gods than love and produced a vivid and complex mythology. But Commerson's encomium expresses very well the delight and astonishment which Tahiti almost always inspired in Europeans.

Captain Cook maintained a tolerant, but objective, view of the islanders' behaviour. He noted that they were generally clean, but infested with lice, that they were prone to steal anything they could lay their hands on, that they were exceedingly hospitable and kind. He strove to keep his men from sexually fraternizing with the Tahitian women as much to prevent the primitives from being infected with syphilis as from regard for naval discipline. He was unsuccessful because, as he wryly noted, 'I was not assisted by any one person in the ship.'

It has been said that Christian Europe and pagan Polynesia represent the opposite poles of 'permissiveness'. Danielsson drew up a table comparing the two cultures in terms of their eroticism and the results may be summarized as follows: while the Polynesians were much more permissive about revealing their bodies, about sex generally, and about abortion and infanticide, Europeans allowed more freedom in choice of marriage partners (he was writing in the 1950s). The Polynesians prohibited marriage between people of different classes, and between cousins; they prohibited intercourse during pregnancy, before war or fishing, and between close relatives and people of the same sex (these latter two prohibitions he found both cultures shared).

Most of the Polynesian prohibitions are clearly related to taboo and magic rather than to what we could call morality. On the other hand, lest the degree of voluptuous freedom, already startling by British standards, be too constricting, the Polynesians had certain fixed occasions when 'they went further and treated the existing laws of morality as null and void'. 'Rape' was, Danielsson found, permitted; but it was the expected acquiescence of girls to sexual advances rather than the violent assault conjured up by the word here. This apart, the only permitted activity which would probably shock a sophisticated European is infanticide. Because of the prevailing sexual licence, and ignorance of contraceptive techniques, large numbers of surplus babies were a feature of life on the overcrowded islands. Adoption and communal rearing were two solutions to the problem. Infanticide was accepted as another. Indeed, in the notorious Arioi Society, devoted to dance and sexual displays, it was a condition of membership that all children born to members must be murdered immediately on birth. If this Eden enjoyed social grace and a sexual freedom unimaginable in Europe, it also displayed a shallowness of emotional response and a casual attitude to life and death which are equally alien to our consciousness.

I have, following Danielsson, used the past tense in discussing Polynesian culture, since, as described above, it no longer exists. Indeed, for a time, it was touch and go as to whether any Polynesians at all would survive. They seemed fated, as the Amazonian Indians do today, to perish as a result of contact with Europeans.

The first foreigners to make a strong impact on Polynesian life were unscrupulous deserters from the ships. Such men were often criminals. They encouraged the Polynesian women to participate in extravagant sexual orgies and, within a few decades, prostitution, hitherto unknown, was flourishing in the islands. As a result, venereal disease, the previous absence of which was undoubtedly a factor in generating the carefree Polynesian attitude towards sexuality, spread alarmingly, as did minor European diseases like measles and influenza which, because the natives had no resistance, proved devastating. By 1830 or thereabouts the population of the islands had been reduced to scarcely one-tenth its original figure.

Other 'gifts' from Europe were drink and firearms which, in their different ways, continued the erosion of the traditional cultures. Finally came the missionaries to systematically complete the dismantling of Polynesian life.

Moerenhout, whose voyages were published in 1837, laments:

> How low this still gentle and friendly people has fallen ... both men and women are nearly always lying down and resting, with dull expressionless eyes ... The most distasteful thing, however, is the complete lack of cleanliness in the houses.

The islands have, by now, recovered their former populations and in fairness it must be added that a new, and vastly more enlightened, generation of missionaries is helping them into the twentieth century. But with the passing of the old Polynesia, the last true Garden of Eden on earth closed down forever.

The chief significance of the expulsion from the Garden of Eden is undoubtedly the exile from our own sexuality. It is of vital significance that Adam and Eve made themselves aprons. They thus divorced themselves forever from unselfconscious genital sexuality and opened the way towards building civilizations out of the sexual energy thus diverted. A good thing or a bad thing? All one can say is that it happened, and try as we might, we can never go back.

THE DISAPPEARING BODY

The human body began to disappear almost as soon as it appeared. It is, in fact, quite likely that the vanishing act started even before fully human creatures arrived. We know that early hominids used tools and it is possible that they used some kind of bodily ornamentation or modification. It is hard to tell because most of these very early 'missing links' are known only from fragmentary fossil remains. In any case, a spear or club is a kind of garment, distinguishing its bearer from animals. Now *homo habilis*, who certainly used weapons and other tools, was probably about four feet tall and had only two-thirds as much brain as modern man.

The fact that he used artefacts and *may* have worn ornaments means the human body was already less than completely natural millions of years before *homo sapiens*, our species, ever emerged.

Indeed, the earliest signs of body modification go back before the hominids, at least insofar as they can be inferred from the behaviour of modern apes. Jane Goodall, in her touching and meticulous account of wild chimpanzee behaviour at Gombe in East Africa, lists nine examples of weapon and tool use. She observed chimpanzees using sticks as weapons or missiles, probing with shorter sticks and straws, using chewed leaves as a sponge and as toilet paper and 'fishing' for termites with straws. She gives no example of wild chimps decorating themselves but Dr. Wolfgang Kohler has observed such behaviour in captive apes; In his book *The Mentality of Apes*, speaking of chimpanzees, he states:

> Almost daily, the animals can be seen walking about with a rope, a
> bit of rag, a blade of grass or a twig on their shoulders ... No

> observer can escape the impression ... [that] the objects hanging
> about the body serve the function of *adornment* ...

Other observers have seen apes wearing newspaper that has blown into their cages and experiments have revealed that apes have a marked colour sense, the females preferring the brighter colours.

There are three chief theories about the origin of clothes. These are that clothes were originally designed for decoration, for modesty or for protection. Now, of course, in civilized societies, these three are often fused. A mink coat, for example, obviously fulfills all three roles. But most authorities today believe that the first function, decoration, is the essential one. This would seem to be supported by the behaviour of the caged apes. There is, however, a fourth contender and this is the 'amulet theory'. According to this interesting theory, the primal origin of clothing must be sought in the wearing of 'life giving substances' such as the red cowrie shells, much used by primitives even today, and found in prehistoric burial sites. The cowrie shell is suggestive of the female genitals. It thus becomes a symbol of what Redgrove and Shuttle call a 'female blood mystery'.

Now apes do not, of course, have any systematized magical beliefs. This would be impossible without language. But Jane Goodall several times witnessed an impressive 'rain dance'. During a tropical thunderstorm she saw female and young chimpanzees perched like spectators in trees while the mature males charged repeatedly down a slope, shaking trees, tearing off huge boughs and dragging them. From her account, it is hard to escape the feeling that some kind of propitiatory or defiance ritual was being enacted and that, at this early stage of mental evolution, magic has already entered the world. On another occasion, she witnessed a chimpanzee, seeking dominance in the group, charge his fellows, clashing together empty paraffin tins which made a deafening racket, perhaps in emulation of thunder.

It thus seems that the rudimentary use of objects as both amulets (the branches and paraffin cans) and ornaments (rope, bits of rag etc.) can be found in chimpanzees. Magic and narcissism seem to be equally primal. Now, of course, a magical shell can also be a pretty shell. Amulet and ornament probably began to fuse psychologically virtually as soon as they were adopted.

Body modification may even precede the use of foreign substances, although the observed behaviour of chimpanzees, as described above, makes one cautious about asserting this positively.

J.C. Flügel, in his admirable study, written from a Freudian point of view, *The Psychology of Clothes* lists five forms of body modification. These are cicatrization (or scarification), tattooing, painting, mutilation, and deformation. With the exception of painting, which requires little more than patience, every one of these alterations of body surface or structure is painful and necessitates what may amount to a hellish ordeal.

In *Down Among the Wild Men*, John Greenway describes circumcision among the Australian aborigines:

> The boy is laid across their [male relatives'] backs, another relative holds the penis and the subincision is made ... whoever does it must be a professional – one slip of the knife and the boy bleeds to death. The stone knife slits the penis from meatus to scrotum. No restraint is put on the boy, and he mustn't show any sign of pain beyond a silent grimace. When it is over, he is a man. It is about the worst ordeal a human male can imagine and nothing can frighten him again.

Mutilation is so widespread that it can almost be considered universal. The reason for this is that some form of circumcision is very widely practised throughout the world. Male circumcision is, indeed, still prevalent, without much medical basis, in the most civilized countries. Among primitives, it may take the horrific form described above or it may be chiefly symbolic as with the Polynesians. Female circumcision is quite common too. This often takes the form of removal of the clitoris. This painful tampering with the genital organs is usually connected with initiation ceremonies and signifies the 'coming of age' of the individual.

In addition to circumcision, a large variety of mutilations is found, from holes in the ears, lips and cheeks to the removal of finger-joints or teeth. Often the mutilation requires the use of a foreign object. Plates are inserted into ears and lips. Bones or sticks are jabbed through cheeks, noses, lips, penises. Jewels are lodged in the cheek or nose. Tribal custom, whether or not of magical origin, seems to know few limits in its ruthless attitude to the human body.

Scarification is a form of surface mutilation. The deliberate cuts are usually made to the face but may also be applied to the buttocks or some other part of the body. Afterwards lime or another substance may be rubbed into the fresh wounds to intensify them and ensure durable and prominent scars. The cuts may be simply light symmetrical slashes on either cheek or highly elaborate patterns covering virtually the entire face. This form of body modification was practised by nearly all the aboriginal peoples of Australia and Tasmania, throughout most of Africa south of the Sahara, in pockets in the Americas, and elsewhere. It was performed on both sexes, which distinguishes its use among primitives from its last survival in civilized nations, the German students' sabre-duelling scars which were supposed to give proof of valour and virility. It is possible that the combination of scarification with intensifying substances, or with separate body-painting, paved the way towards tattooing. This would tend to be confirmed by the geographic distribution of these forms of body modification. They are not often found together and, generally speaking, tattooing is more common among relatively more sophisticated peoples who might easily have gone through a scarification and painting phase.

The third and last of what might be termed the 'ordeal' types of body modification is deformation. This is the most repellent of the three since, in some of its manifestations at least, it can result in functional impairment of the body. This was certainly the case with the age-long Chinese practice of binding women's feet. The purpose was to produce a very small foot, and the long-lost motive for this was tied up with the equation of foot size with genital size. There is, in fact, absolutely no scientific basis for equating genital size, either male or female, with the dimensions of any other part of the body, but such equations are regularly made by primitives. Because men are supposed to prize small female genitals, generation after generation of Chinese women had their feet bound so firmly that many were crippled for life, in an attempt to magically ensure genital tightness, or at least to compel belief in it.

Even more upsetting, but mercifully a very localized phenomenon, was the treatment of the wives of one African king. Since fatness was considered the chief attribute of beauty (an equation often made since fatness indicates prosperity and demonstrates sheer spatial magnificence), these poor ladies were fattened like pigs to the point where they could no longer keep their grossly obese bodies erect and had to spend their lives sprawled like pregnant sows on the floors of their huts.

Another form of deformation is the African practice of head-binding to produce ultimately what is an almost horizontal rather than a vertical head, stretching from the chin in front (rather than at bottom) to the crown of the head at the back (rather than at the top). Curious as the results are, there is no evidence that this form of deformation harms either the mental or the functional capacities of the individual.

Lest we be tempted into feelings of superiority to these benighted primitives, it is just as well to remember that Western clothing has never been, and still is not, conspicuous for its sane and healthy qualities. Indeed, thanks to the tight lacing of the waist which was so fashionable until the early twentieth century, it used to be assumed that it was natural for women to breathe from the chest, rather than, like men, from the abdomen. There is of course, absolutely no difference between the breathing of a man and that of an 'undeformed' woman.

We have not included tattooing among the 'ordeal' body modifications and, correctly applied by modern electric-needle techniques, it is not one. But Melville's *Typee* describes an operation performed by traditional techniques in the Marquesas in the early nineteenth century: 'I beheld a man extended flat upon his back on the ground, and despite the forced composure of his countenance, it was evident that he was suffering agony.' Certainly, tattooing among primitives may assume the proportions of an ordeal. Moreover, its consequences can be horrific. Berchon, a French naval surgeon, listed the following complications which he observed during the South Pacific campaign in 1853: pain; ulcerating sores; inflammation, leading to erysipelas, accompanied by fever, leading possibly to death; gangrene, often sufficiently severe to necessitate amputation; the accidental inoculation of disease.

The last of these is still a hazard in modern tattooing parlours and in England and America there are periodic outbreaks of serum hepatitis associated with a specific tattooing parlour. In former times, syphilis could be contracted in this way. For all that, tattooing should not be regarded as intrinsically an ordeal. Performed by a skilled craftsman, with simple or sophisticated techniques, it should be quite bearable and the pain is incidental rather than intrinsic to the operation.

The appeal of tattooing seems to be well-nigh universal. This is not to say that all peoples are tattooed and indeed, as mentioned above, in those areas today where primitives indulge in scarification and body painting it is relatively rare. It is nonetheless found in all parts of the world and must have been independently invented many times. It is of great antiquity. There is evidence that it was used before 8000 BC and it is still flourishing today. Its results can be bewildering, dramatic, witty or, in the case of modern Japanese tattooing, aesthetically delightful. When heavily tattooed natives were first brought to Europe they created a sensation in social circles.

Scutt and Gotch, in their definitive work on the subject, *Skin Deep*, say that 'the reasons for having it done are enigmatic', and then list fourteen! These include camouflage, magical motives, money-making and the registration of important personal medical data, such as blood group. They do not mention the sinister 'Auschwitz' tattoos, a form of branding which enabled the methodical SS to keep track of its intended victims.

Body painting is also very widely practised and very ancient. It survives in civilized communities chiefly in the form of female cosmetics. Unlike the other forms of body modification, painting is temporary. Scutt and Gotch suggest that tattooing might in its origins have been a deliberate attempt to render permanent the camouflage effects of painting. Certain tribes, especially in South America, have elevated body, and especially face, painting to the level of high art and indeed devoted much of their time to its application and reapplication.

All these forms of body modification are clearly related to decoration. They are also undoubtedly related to magic, which may be psychologically more important to primitives. There is, however, a motive for body modification which is rarely discussed. Scutt and Gotch when listing people's memories of how they felt about being tattooed ended with '*the satisfaction of a new acquisition*'. Body modification, in human communities almost devoid of private property, supplies its recipient with a *possession*. A beautifully tattooed, correctly and impressively scarified or traditionally mutilated body will be just as much a source of pride to a primitive as a lovely home or a new car to a modern. If all one owns is a wardrobe and if that wardrobe is restricted to the scars or tattoos on one's body, these become precious indeed.

Terence Turner, writing in the *New Scientist* for 7 June, 1979, describes the Kayapo Indians of the Amazonian basin.

> A well turned-out adult Kayapo male [has] ... a large lower-lip plug (a saucer-like disc some 6 cm. across), penis sheath (a small cone made of palm leaves covering the glans penis), large holes pierced through the ear lobes from which hang small strings of beads, over-all body paint in red and black patterns, plucked eyebrows, eyelashes and facial hair, and head shaved to a point at the crown with the hair left long at the sides and back.

A hundred years ago, such a man would probably have been dismissed as 'a naked savage'. Turner exhaustively analyses each item of the

Kayapo's apparel and body modification and concludes that the man 'is as fully covered in a fabric of cultural meaning as the most elaborately draped Victorian lady or gentleman'.

Almost all the attributes of civilized clothing can be located in combinations of body-modification and simple adornment. The body, the functional, unaltered body, of a monkey or an antelope has already been left far behind. And the two remaining motives for the wearing of clothes – protection and modesty, have not as yet even been touched upon.

Protection can be divided into two categories: protection from natural and from supernatural hazards. Undoubtedly, for primitives, the latter is more important and this is amply catered for by the mystical significance of some forms of body modification. What of physical protection? It undoubtedly plays a part in the origin and development of clothing but a much less important one than is generally supposed. Various observers have pointed out that the actual clothing worn throughout the world is more traditional than function-al, and often serves as a very ineffective defence against either cold or heat. The inhabitants of Tierra del Fuego lived naked in a bitter climate, and there are other examples of similar contempt for weather or climate. True, in high or arctic regions, protective clothing is indispensable but elsewhere on the earth, protection from weather seems to be at most an ancillary reason for the practice of wearing clothes.

Now to modesty. A pious Victorian would certainly have assumed that the chief purpose of clothing is to conceal 'the shameful parts'. It is, of course, not nearly as simple as that. Clothing, as we have already seen, is very intimately connected with all the physical and psycho-logical attributes of man. For this reason, generalizations are danger-ous. There is no consistency of motive or practice. Nevertheless, it would be nearer the truth to say that one important purpose of clothing is to emphasize the body rather than to conceal it. Certainly, among primitives, almost all adornment, or rudimentary concealment, of the genitals is for the purpose of drawing attention to them rather than hiding them. There are tribes in which only the prostitutes are clothed. The men of Pongo in French West Africa refused to allow their women to be clothed because this would immediately make them *more* seductive. Modesty, it is probably fair to say, in the sense of hiding the 'shameful parts' develops only after the habitual use of clothing. It is almost certain that modesty played a negligible part in the evolution of clothes.

The increasing complexity and/or subtlety of clothing, throughout the civilized ages, has almost certainly been a function of the increasing complexity of life in general. Human beings have become more mobile which means they have needed greater versatility in their clothing. They have acquired more and more material possessions and items as various as money and weapons have required support from clothes. They have developed more and more elaborate social and political systems which have generated specialized clothes like uniforms and others related to the demands of a craft or trade. They have become wealthier, and rich and abundant apparel is one of the most self-aggrandizing, and therefore pleasurable, ways of displaying wealth. Clothes need not, of course, be ostensibly magnificent in order to indicate status. One of the most compelling ways of displaying wealth, as people have increasingly decided in this century, is to refrain from displaying it at all. Thus, for instance, the 'little black dress' may be the ultimate garment in a well-dressed woman's wardrobe, and duchesses sport jeans. Obviously, the potential of the varying textures, colours and shapes of clothes is enormous, greatly transcending even those offered by painting or tattooing. Clothes are also used to expand and modify the shape of the body in ways which can lead to ludicrous excesses. One Venetian courtesan wore a kind of stilted boot which raised her so high and made her footing so precarious that she could only walk abroad with a companion on each side to support her. Trains, for the purpose of increasing size, can get so large (as in the celebrated coronation robe of Catherine II of Russia) that the women ostensibly bearing them disappear in a kind of landscape of fabric. The fashionable excesses of female clothes have long been ridiculed. Rudofsky wittily designed, and had made for him by Constantino Nivola, a series of four plaster figures showing what the female body would be like if its shape was really the one suggested by a particular fashion. Thus the lady in a bustle becomes a quadruped, a kind of squashed-up centaur.

But, invariably, the sexual motif re-emerges in clothing. Flügel has demonstrated how items of clothing not only increase the allure of both sexes but 'may themselves actually symbolize the sexual organs'. Shoes, ties, hats, collars, even coats, trousers and capes, may be phallic symbols while shoes, jewels, girdles and garters may be symbols of female genitals. Certainly the erotic parts of the body are the focal points of all fashion. As female hem lines rise and fall, neck lines

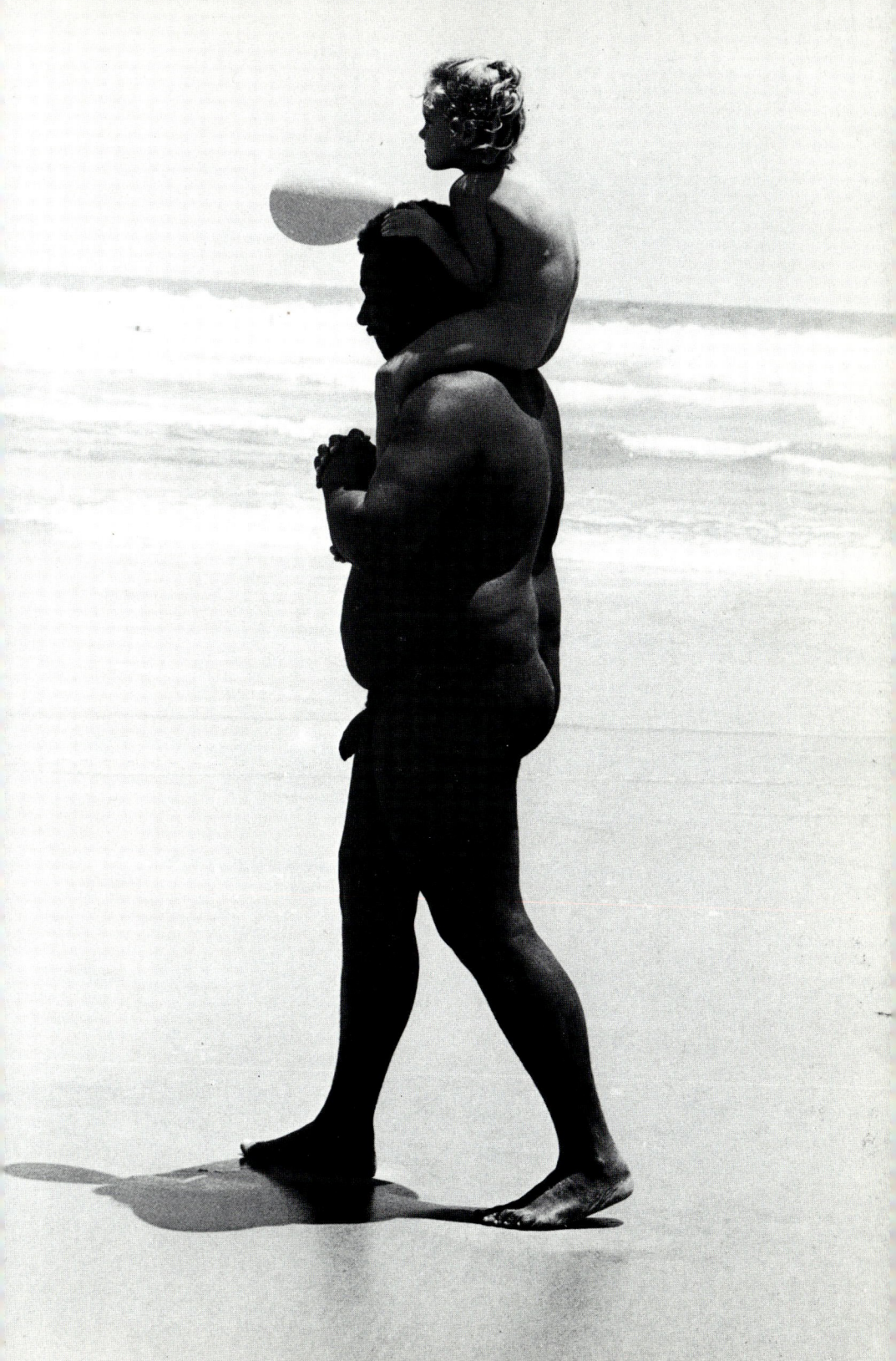

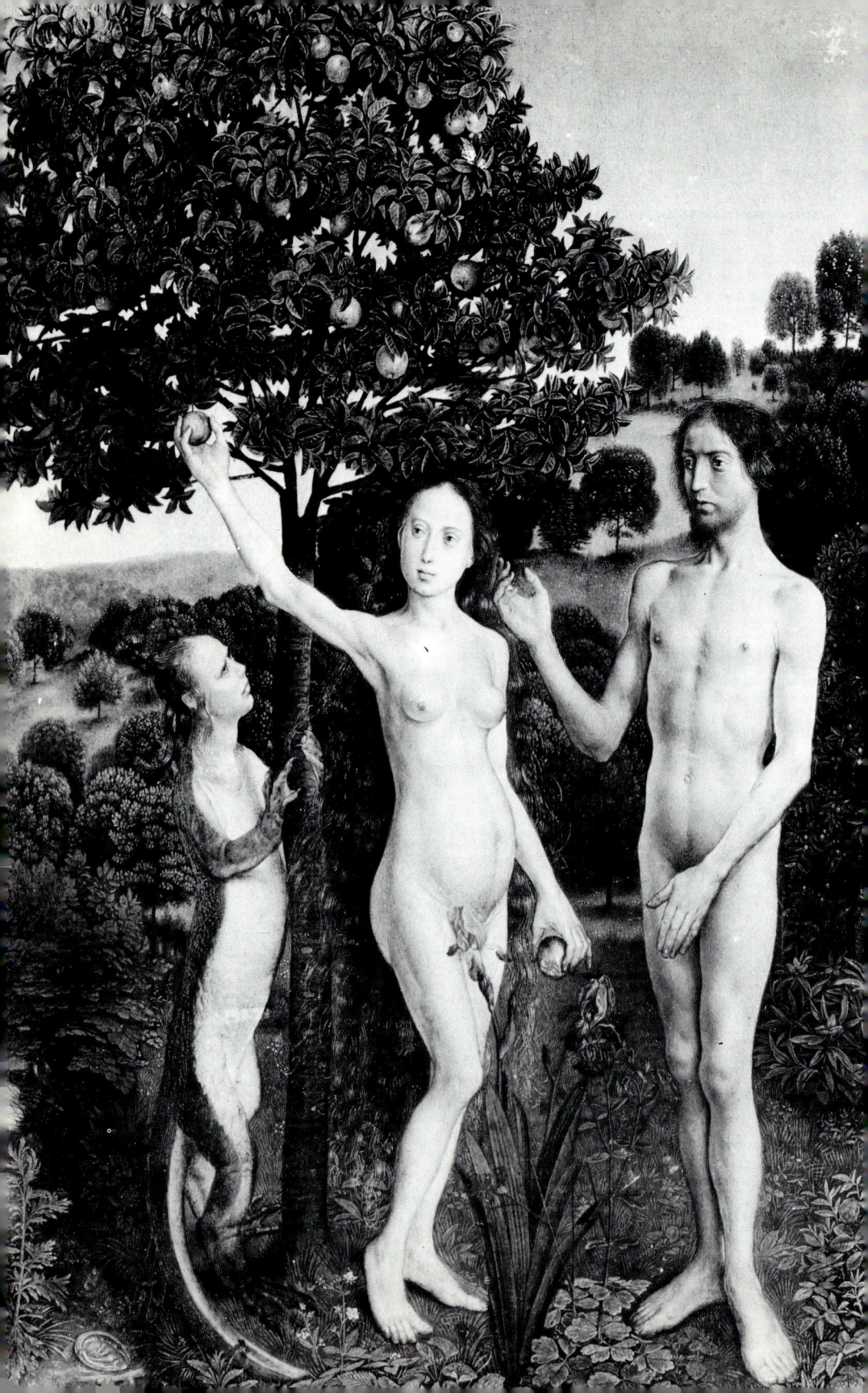

Naked in the Garden of Eden, Adam and Eve were neither evil nor good; like animals, they existed in an amoral state that precedes the generation of good or evil. In this painting of *The Fall* by Hugo van der Goes (left), the serpent's face shows him to be basically equal to the human inhabitants of the Garden. Only after Adam and Eve's discovery of a moral view of the universe was the serpent reduced to ground level. Yet even today there are people who live in conditions similar to those in the Garden of Eden. Cooperation with nature, rather than an attempt to dominate it, is a characteristic of the life-style of the Indians of the upper waters of the Amazon (below). The giant figleaf of Mack Sennett's bathing beauty (right), though meant to be funny, still symbolizes the ambiguous labyrinth of human morality and civilization.

(Previous page) A modern return to Eden? A scene on a nudist beach in California.

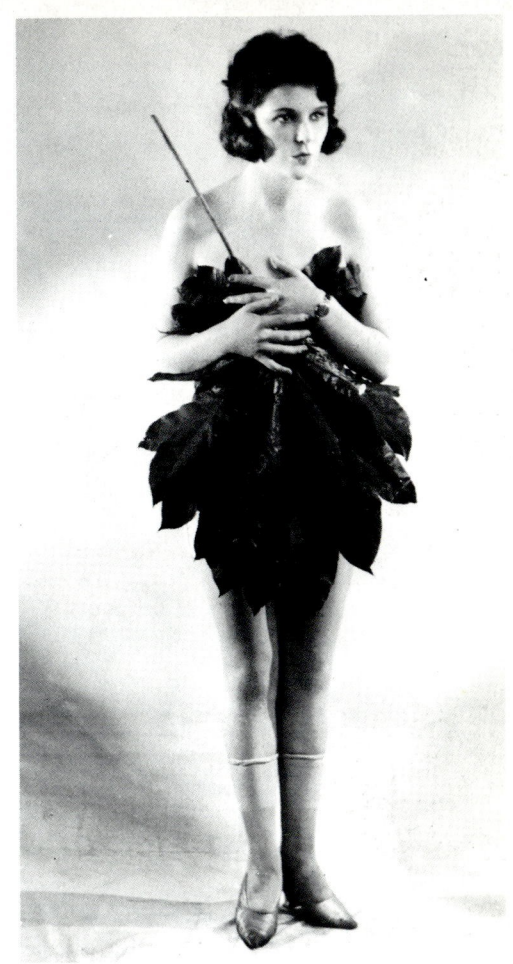

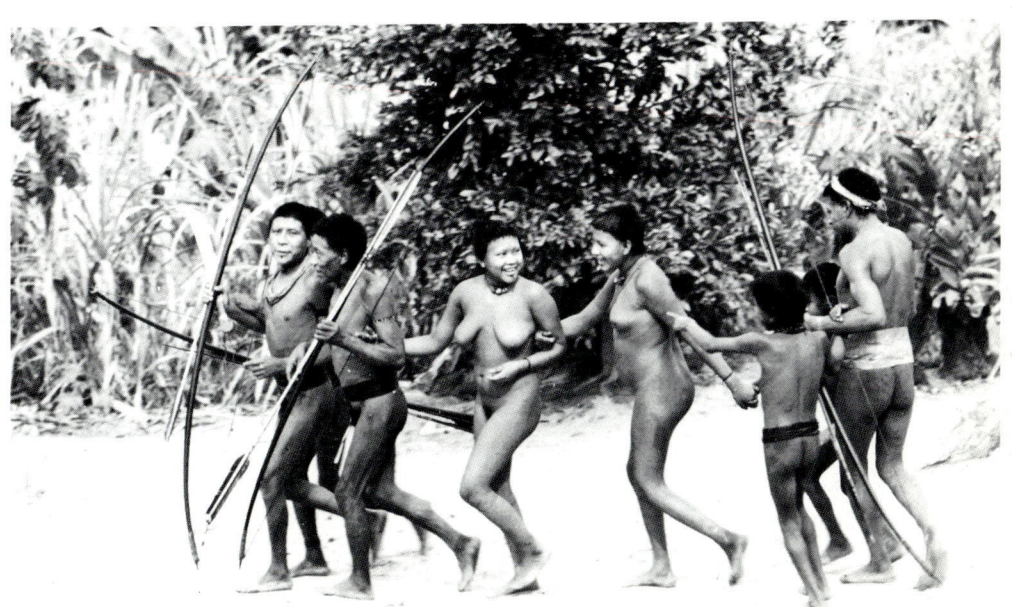

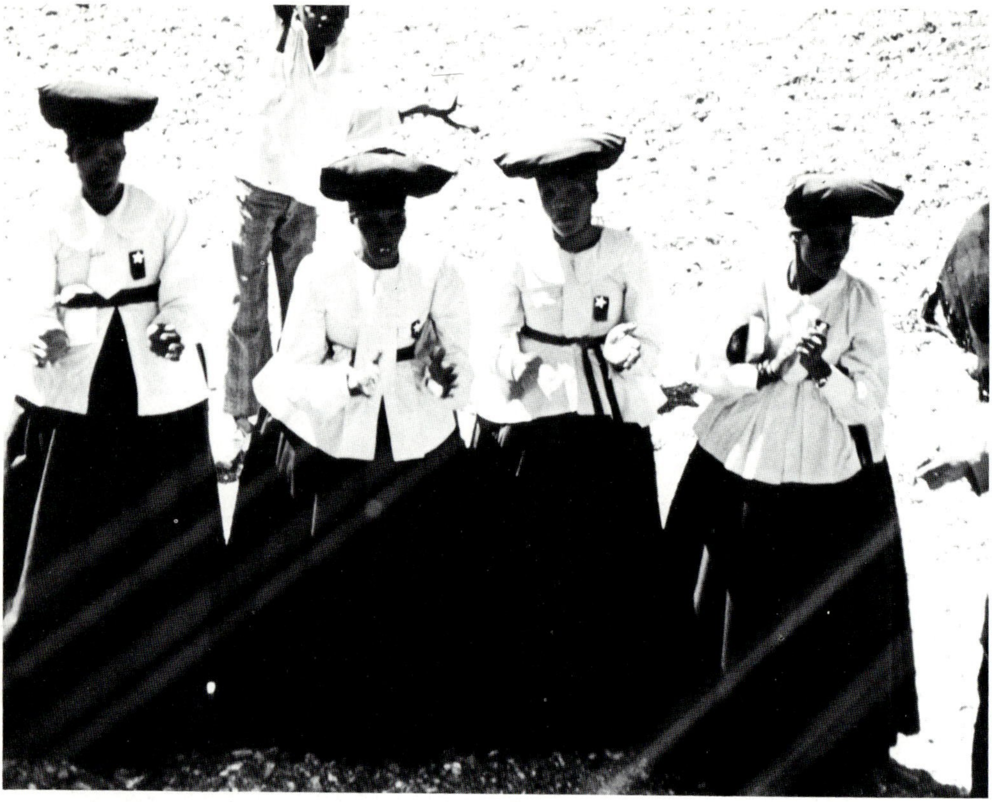

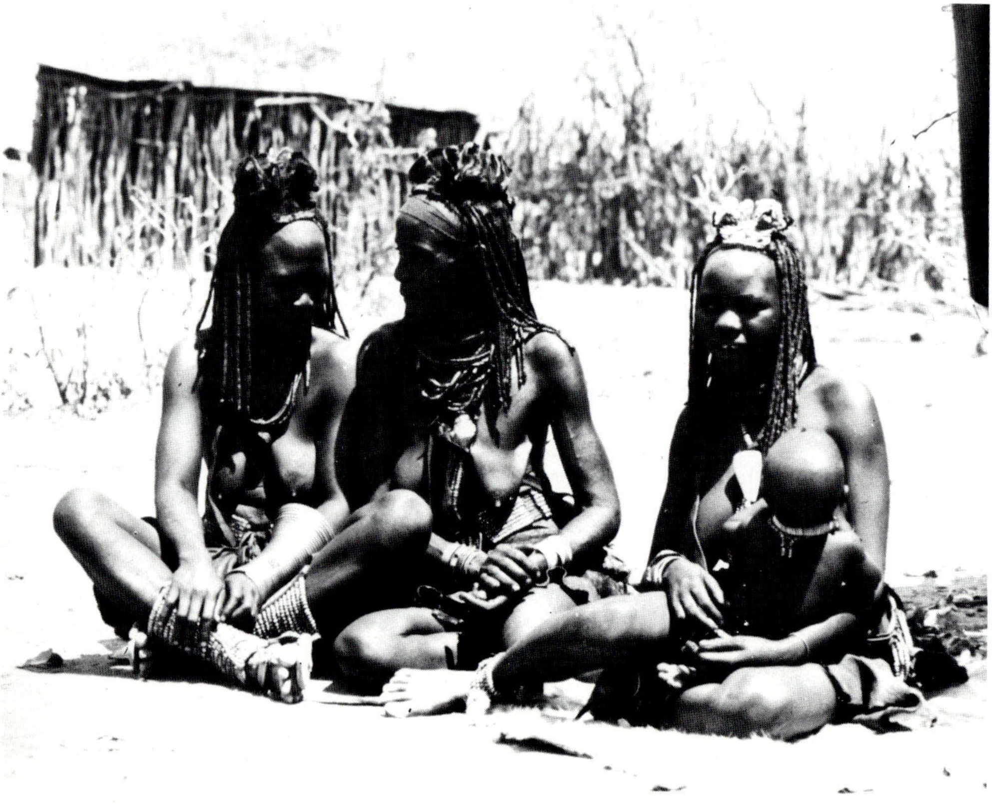

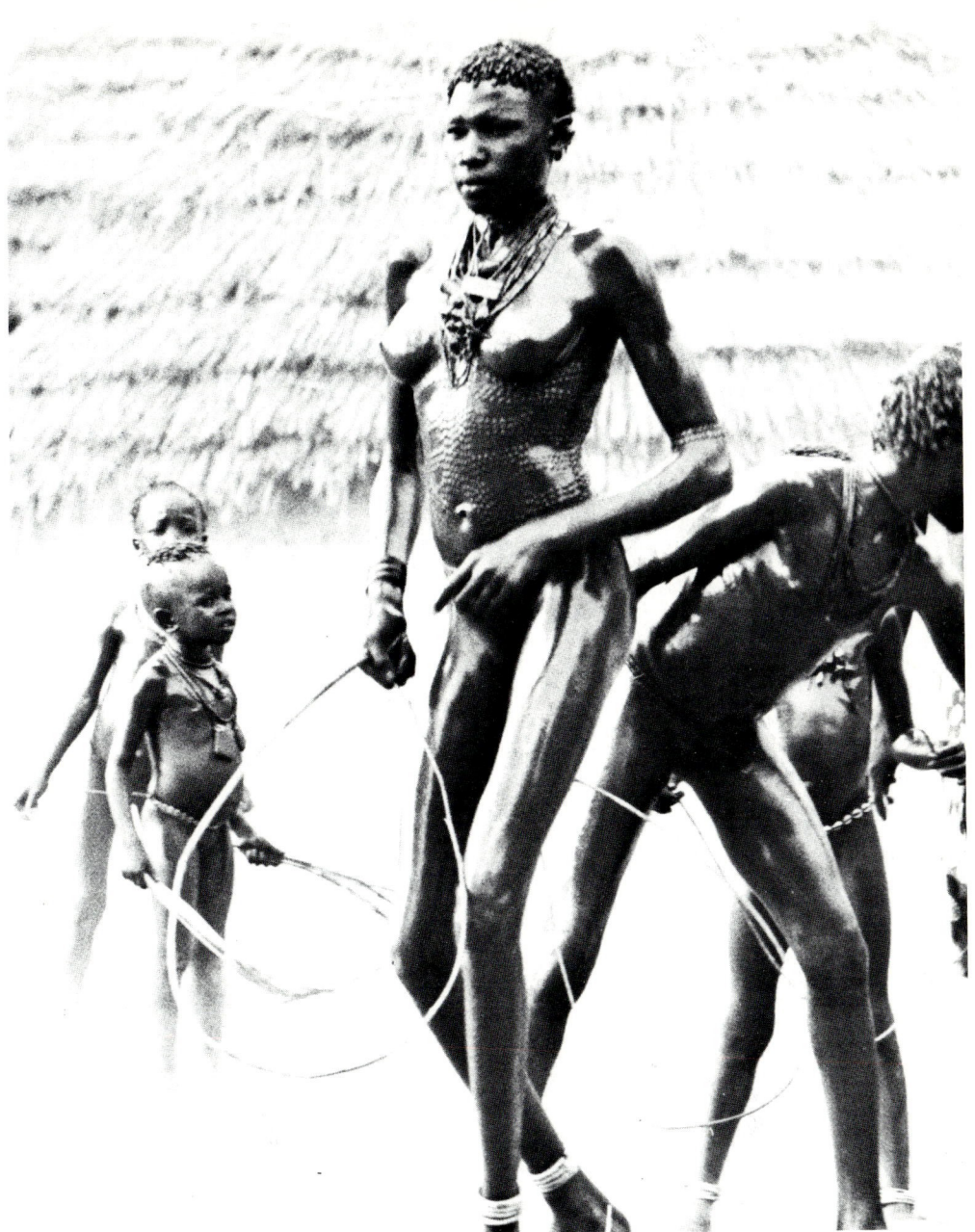

Children in naked cultures do not grow up in ignorance of sex. Even the youngest can take part in this erotically exciting dance of love among the girls of the northern Sudan (above). It was inevitably displays of this kind that first experienced the reforming zeal of nineteenth century missionaries. A dramatic example of their influence can be seen in the two photographs opposite. Compare the Herero women of Namibia in their natural state (below) with those of the Herero Lutheran Choir (above). However, in clothing the naked, the missionaries were disconcerted to find they had produced, not an improvement in native morals, but a deterioration.

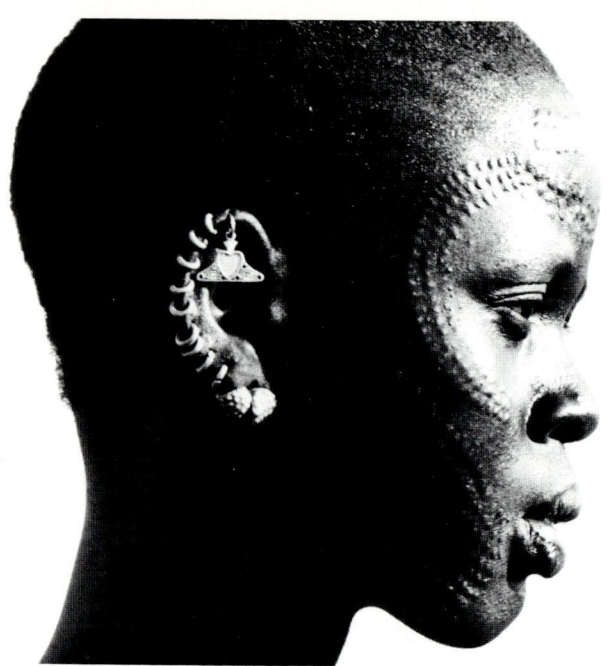

The instinct to decorate predates man. Some of the more primitive types of body modification involve an 'ordeal'. Both men and women may be subjected to circumcision, scarification or deformation. Decoration may vary from delicate and intricate scarification, combined with ear-rings, necklaces, lip-fringes and many other kinds of adornment, to the inserted lip discs of the Nigerian woman (above right) or the decorated penis sheaths of the male (below right).

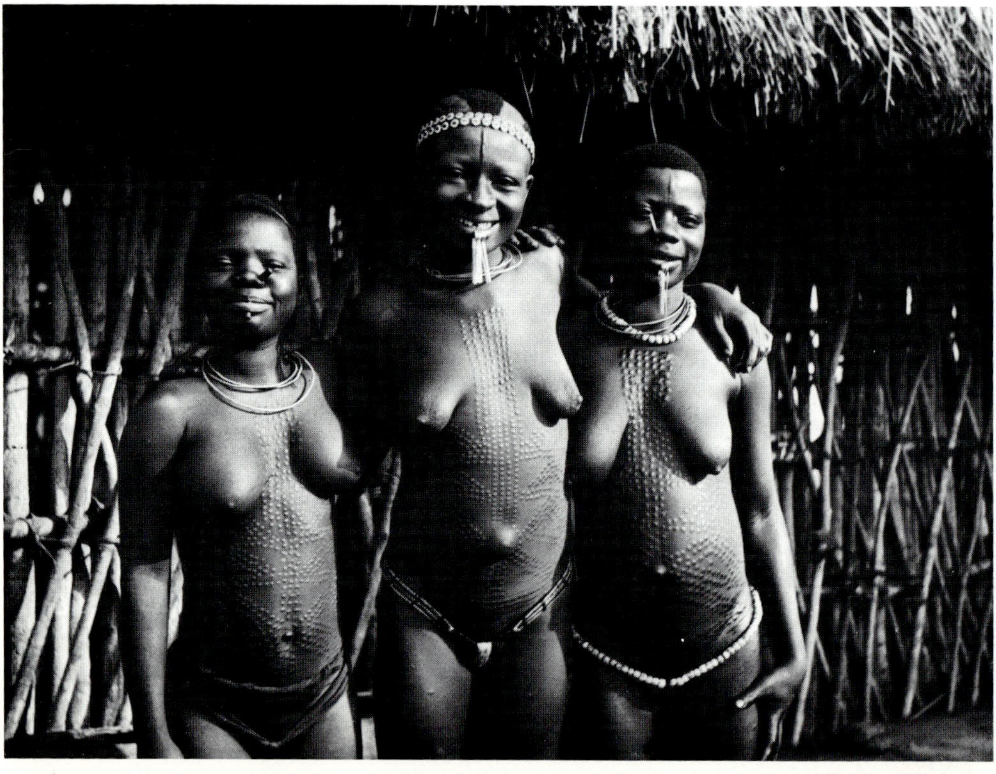

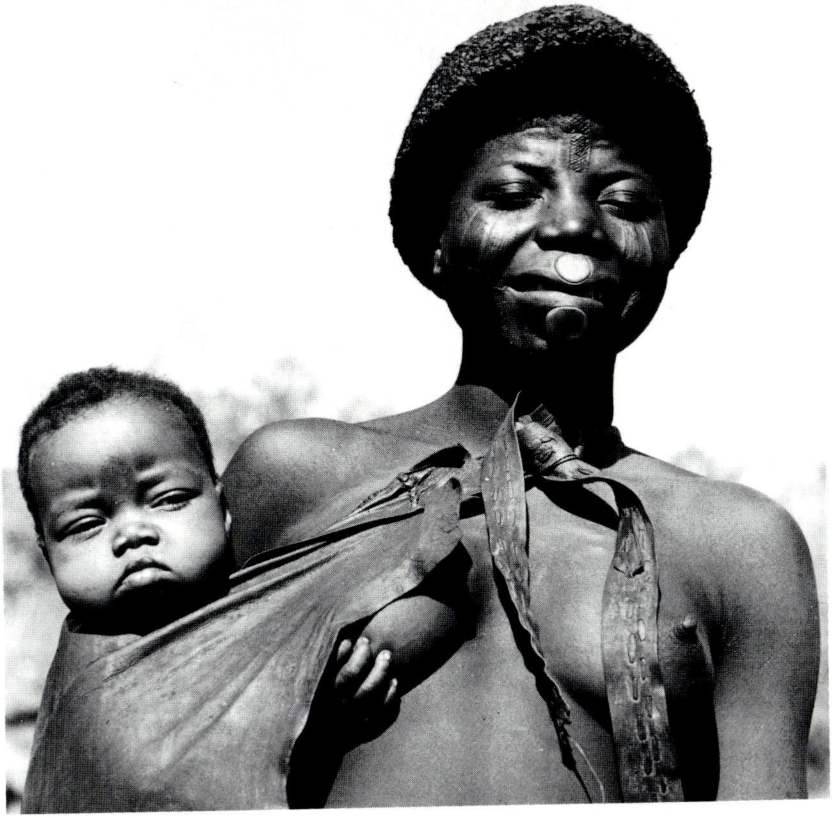

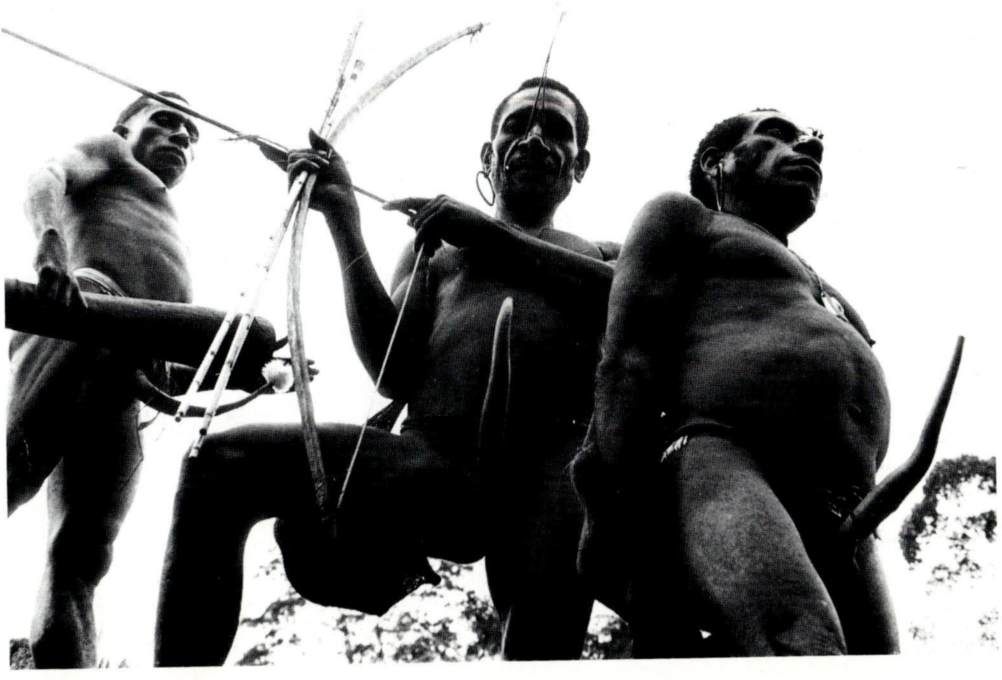

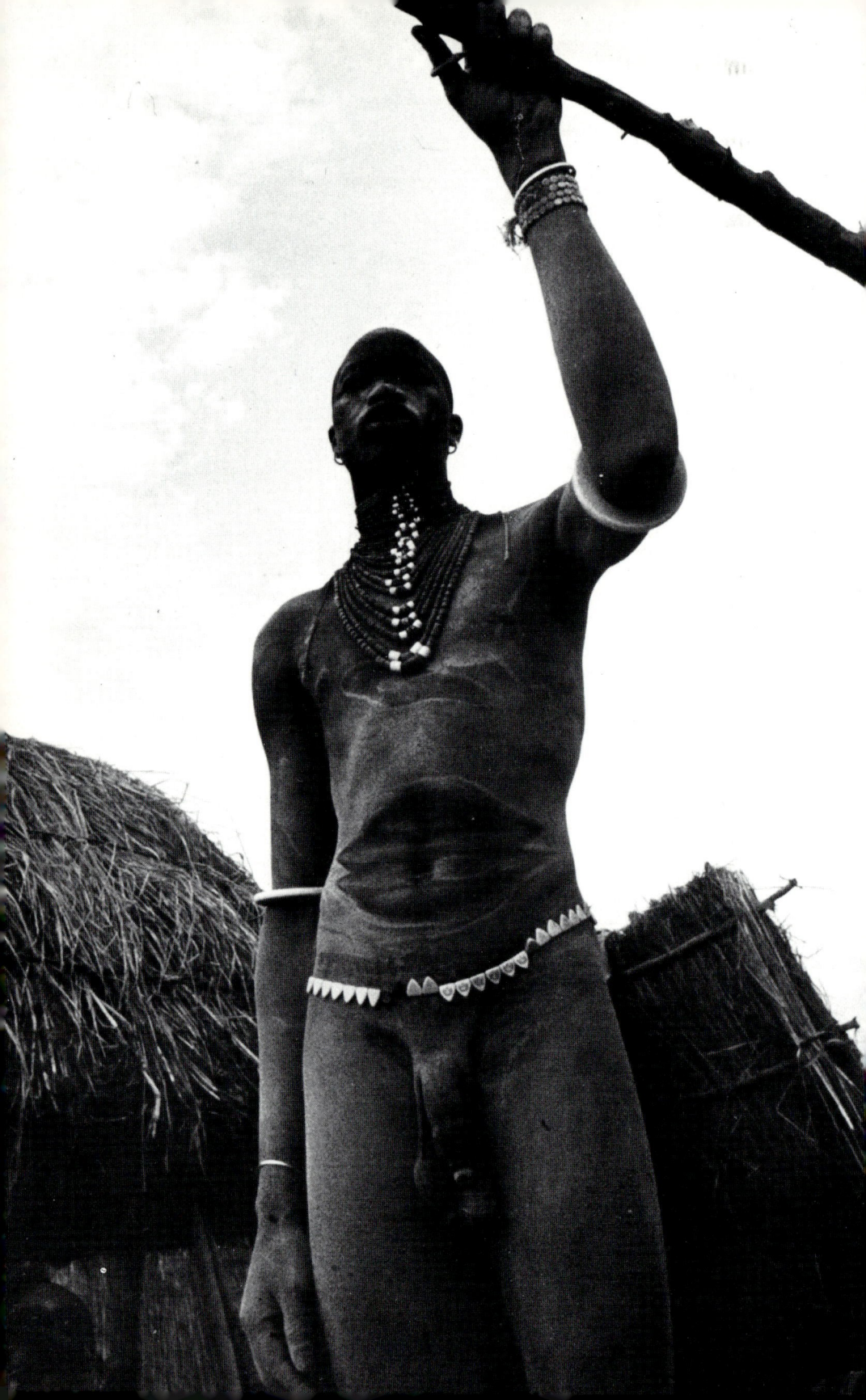

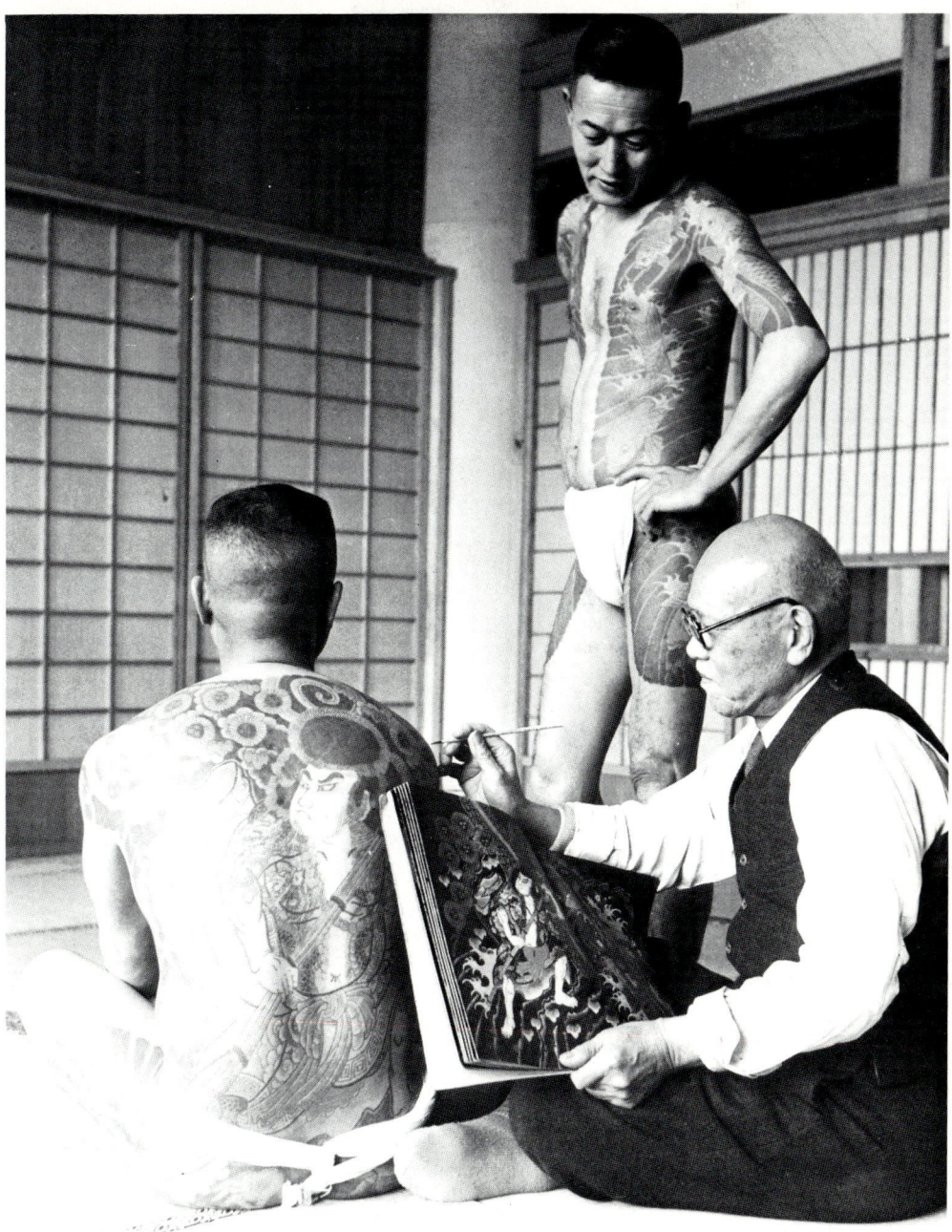

While deep scarification (left) is undoubtedly a test of endurance, tattooing – at least in its modern manifestations – is hardly an 'ordeal', although it can still prove painful and even dangerous. It is found in all parts of the world and appears to be of great antiquity. It can be dramatic, witty or, as in modern Japanese tattooing (above) aesthetically attractive. Many Japanese criminals are today heavily tattooed, both as a defiant gesture against society, and as a sign of common-fellowship.

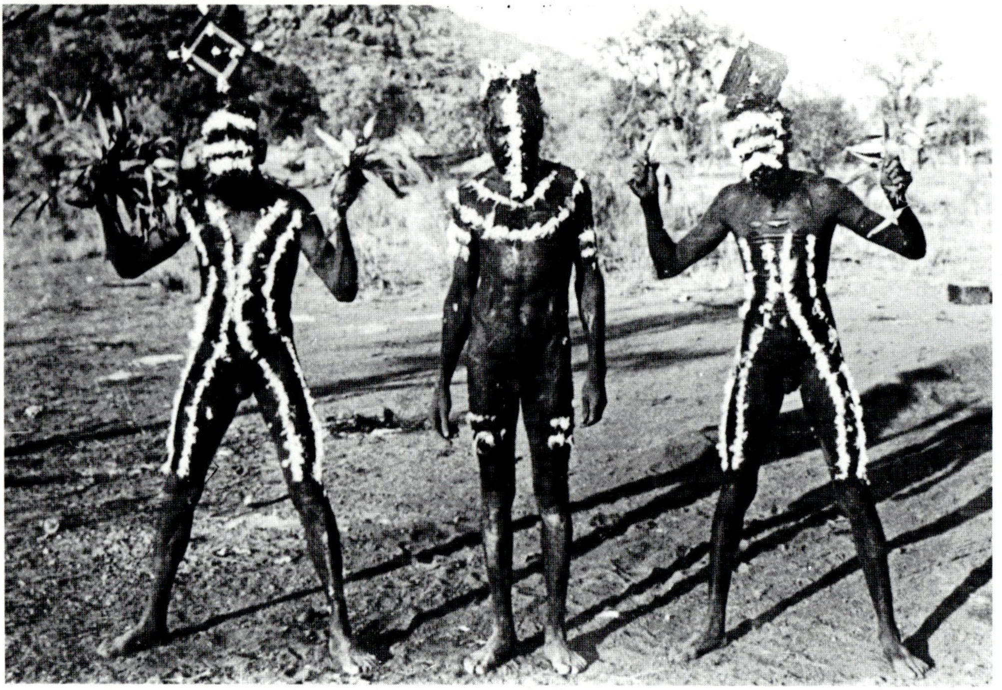

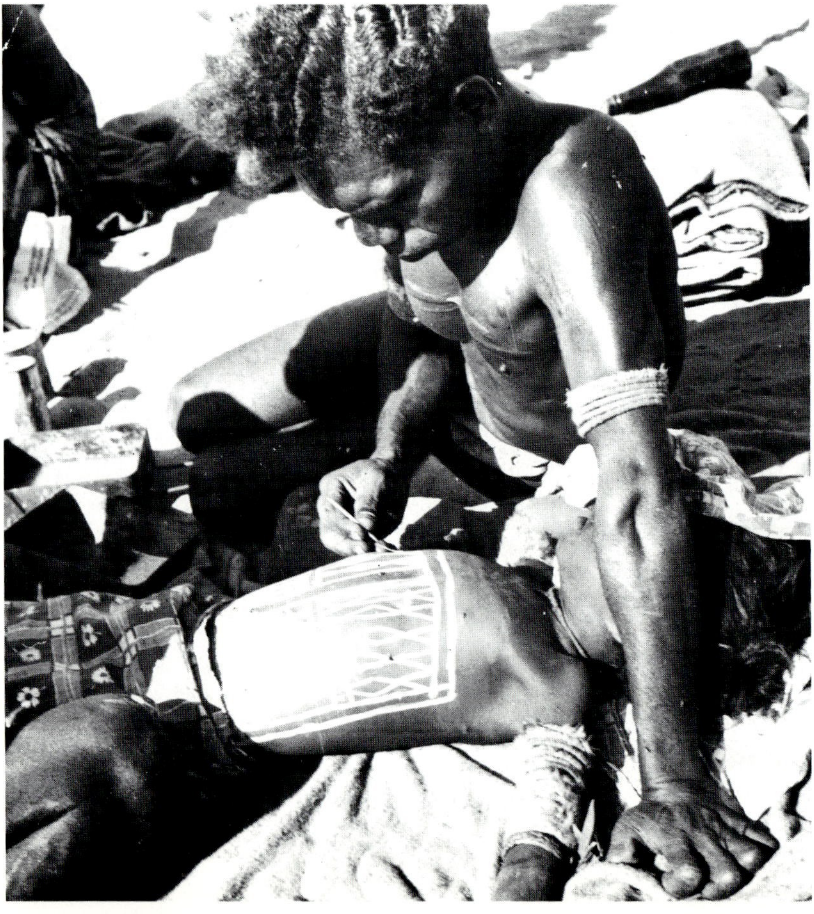

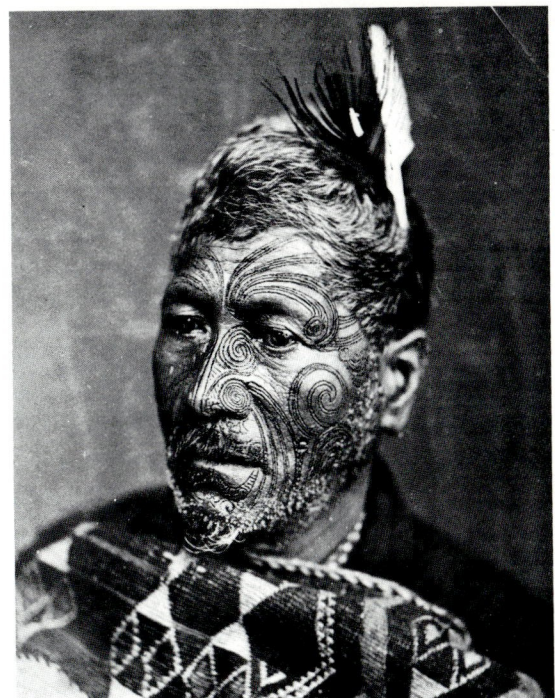

The appeal of abstract patterns of body decoration is universal. Tattooing (above, a Maori chieftain) may have its origins in an attempt to render permanent the effects of body painting. Australian aboriginals practise simple body painting to prepare a boy for circumcision (below left) and sometimes add feathers and other fibres for elaborate initiation ceremonies (above left). Even in the sophisticated west, body painting enjoyed an unexpected revival during the 1960s (below).

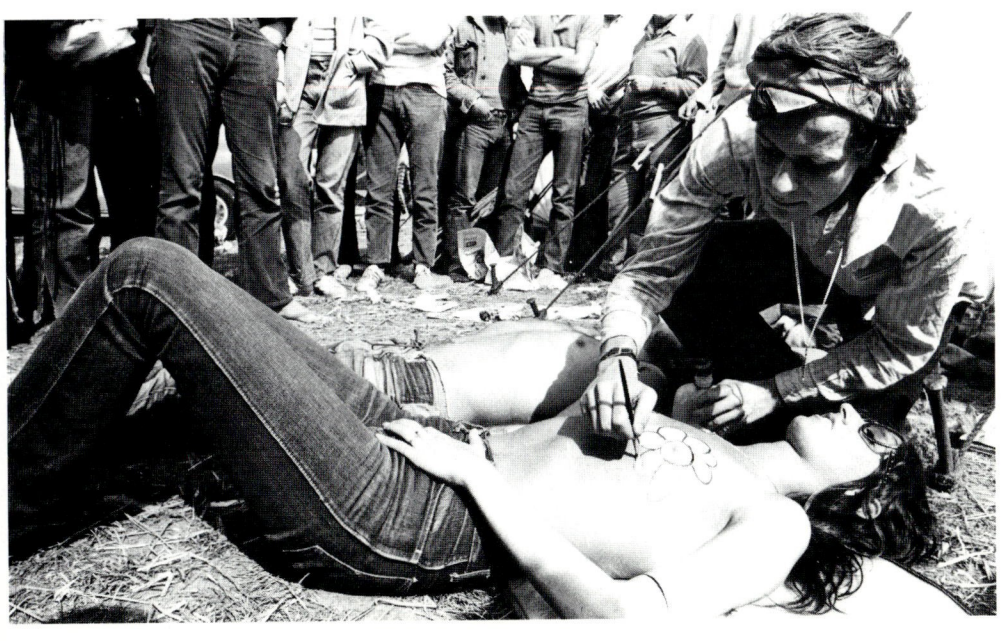

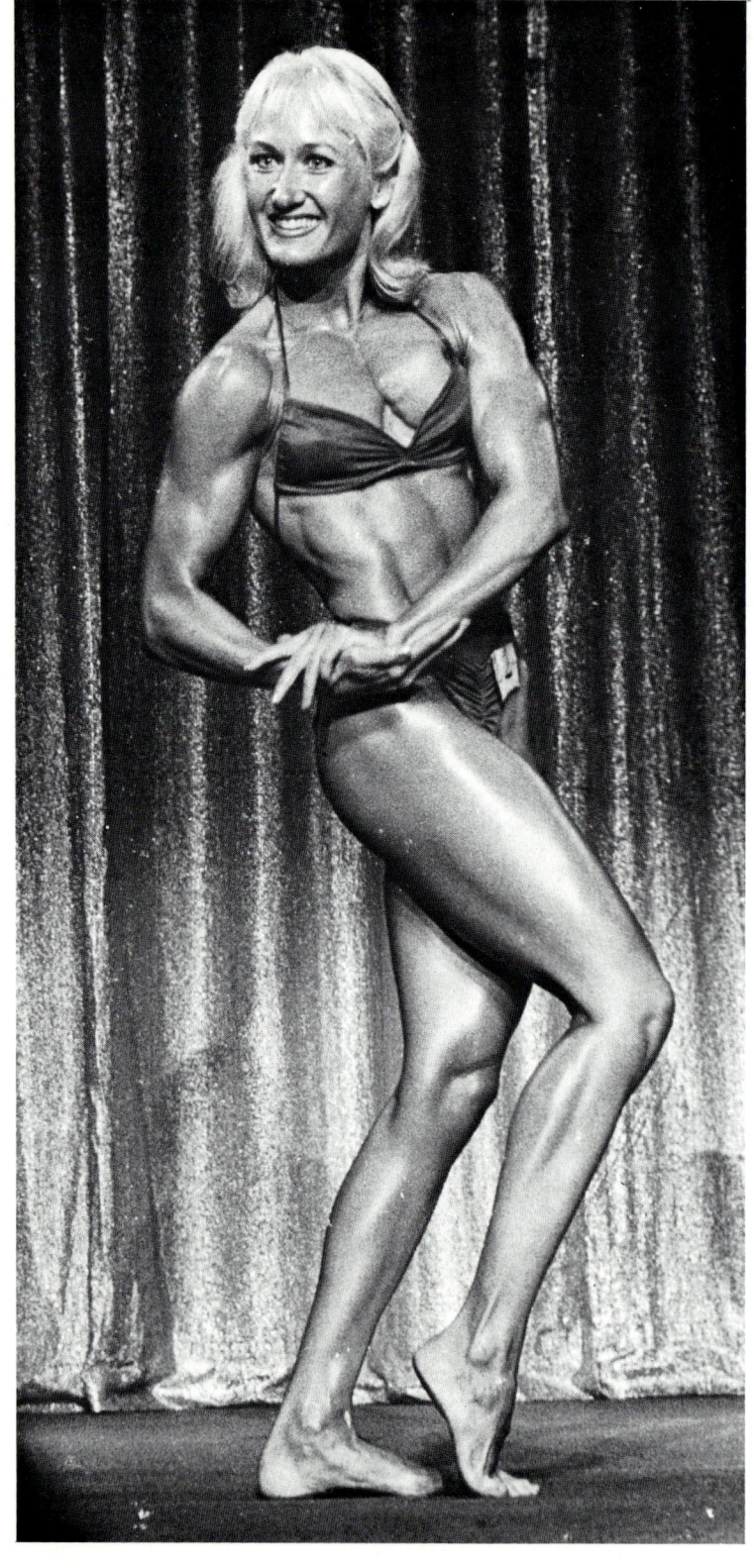

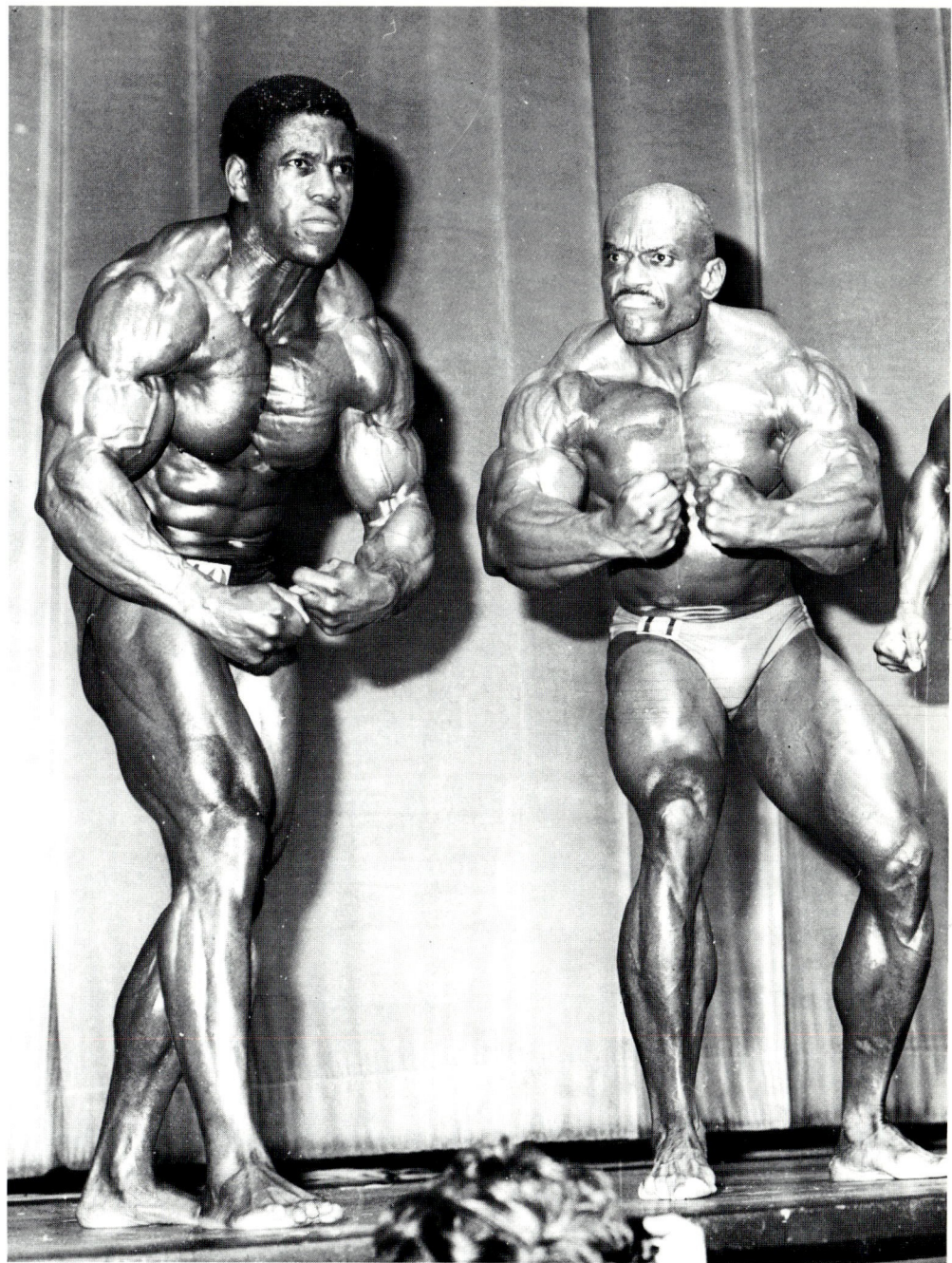

The cult of 'the body beautiful' has led to an obsession with the development of muscle at the expense of the more sensuous contours of the human form. The female body-builder (left) may retain her feminine appeal, but the more extreme examples of male musclemen, nourished on anabolic steroids (above), to many eyes verge on the obscene.

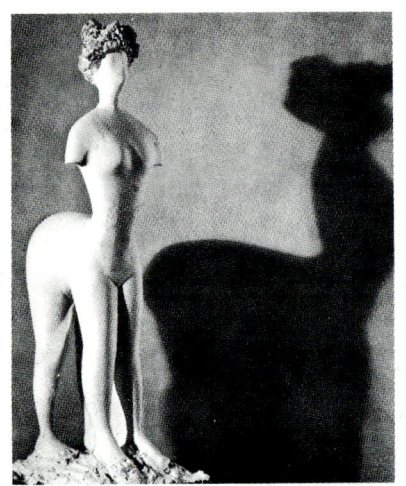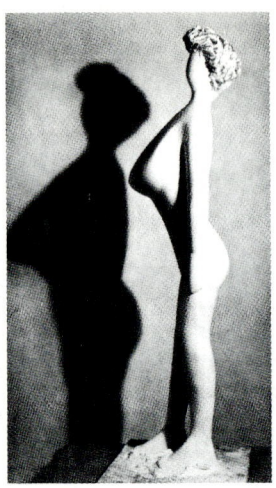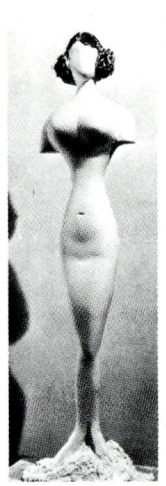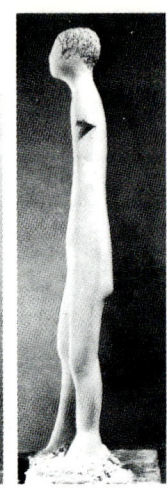

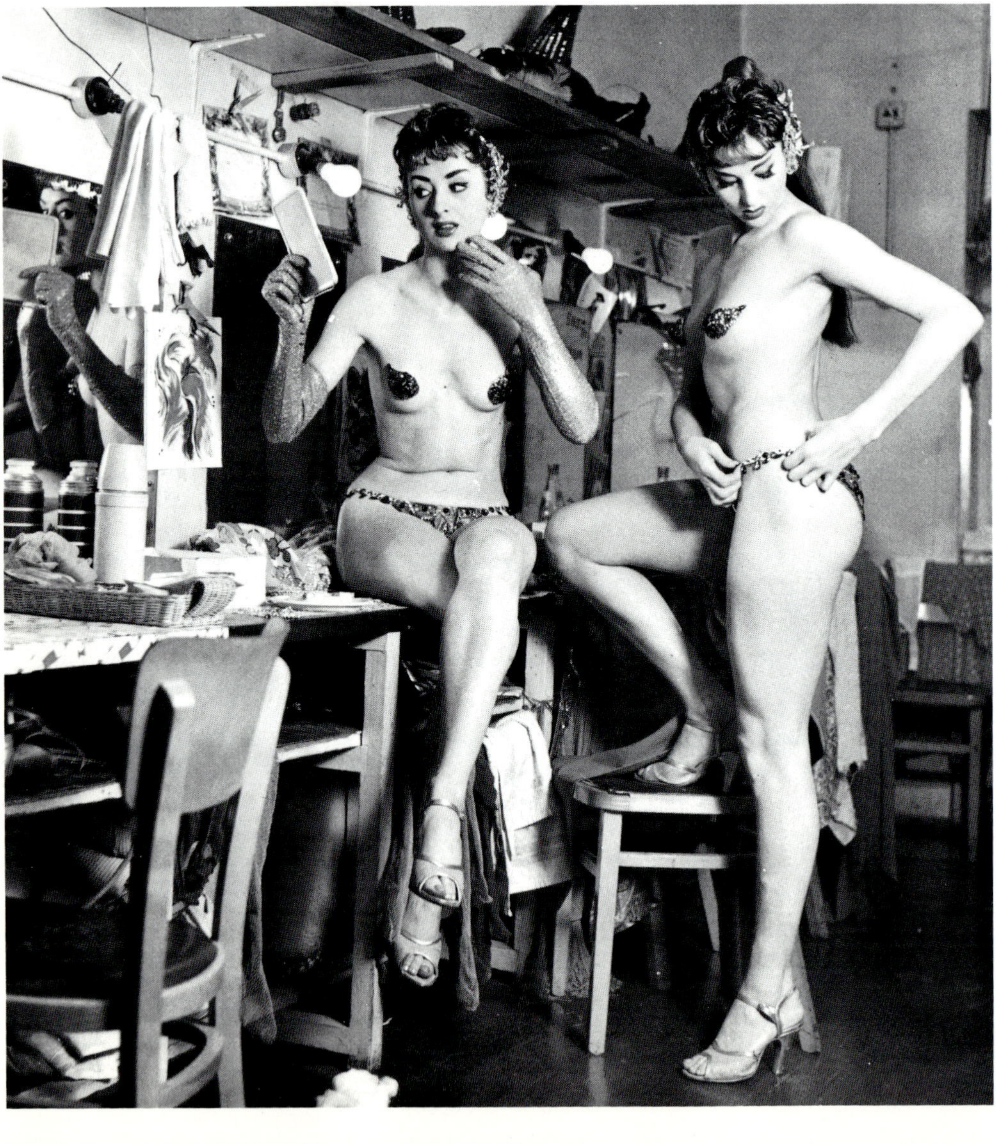

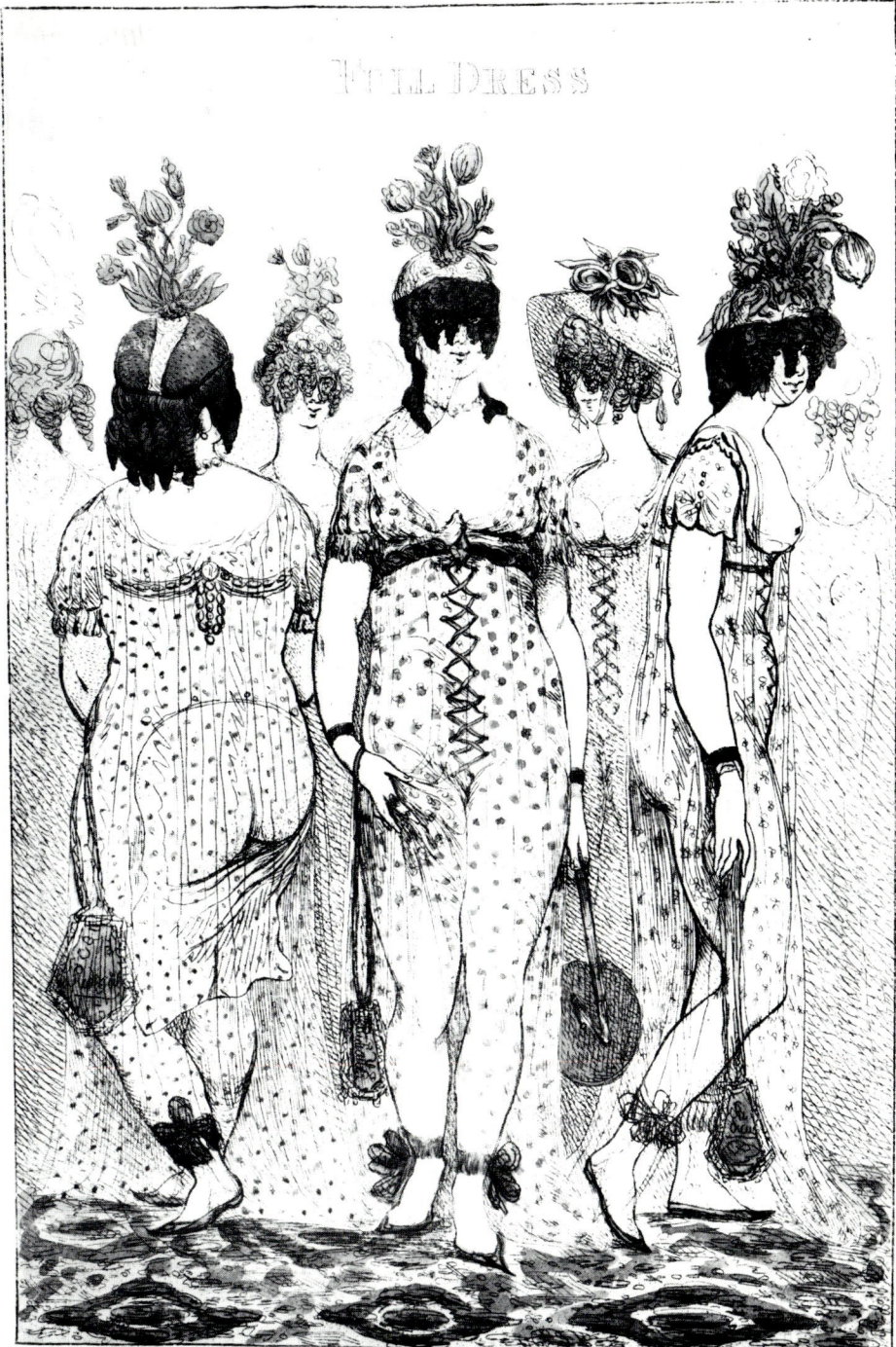

Fashion, more than morality, dictates what parts of the body may be revealed. Rudofsky, in his *Unfashionable Human Body* (modelled by Costantino Nivola, above left) amused himself with imagining what forms of the female body would have produced the fashionable silhouettes of various ages. In 1800, Empire fashions were more concerned with revealing than concealing (above), while in more recent times the question of how much of the areola might be revealed has resulted in the emphasis of the nipples (left). The ultimate development in this direction is the topless dress (overleaf).

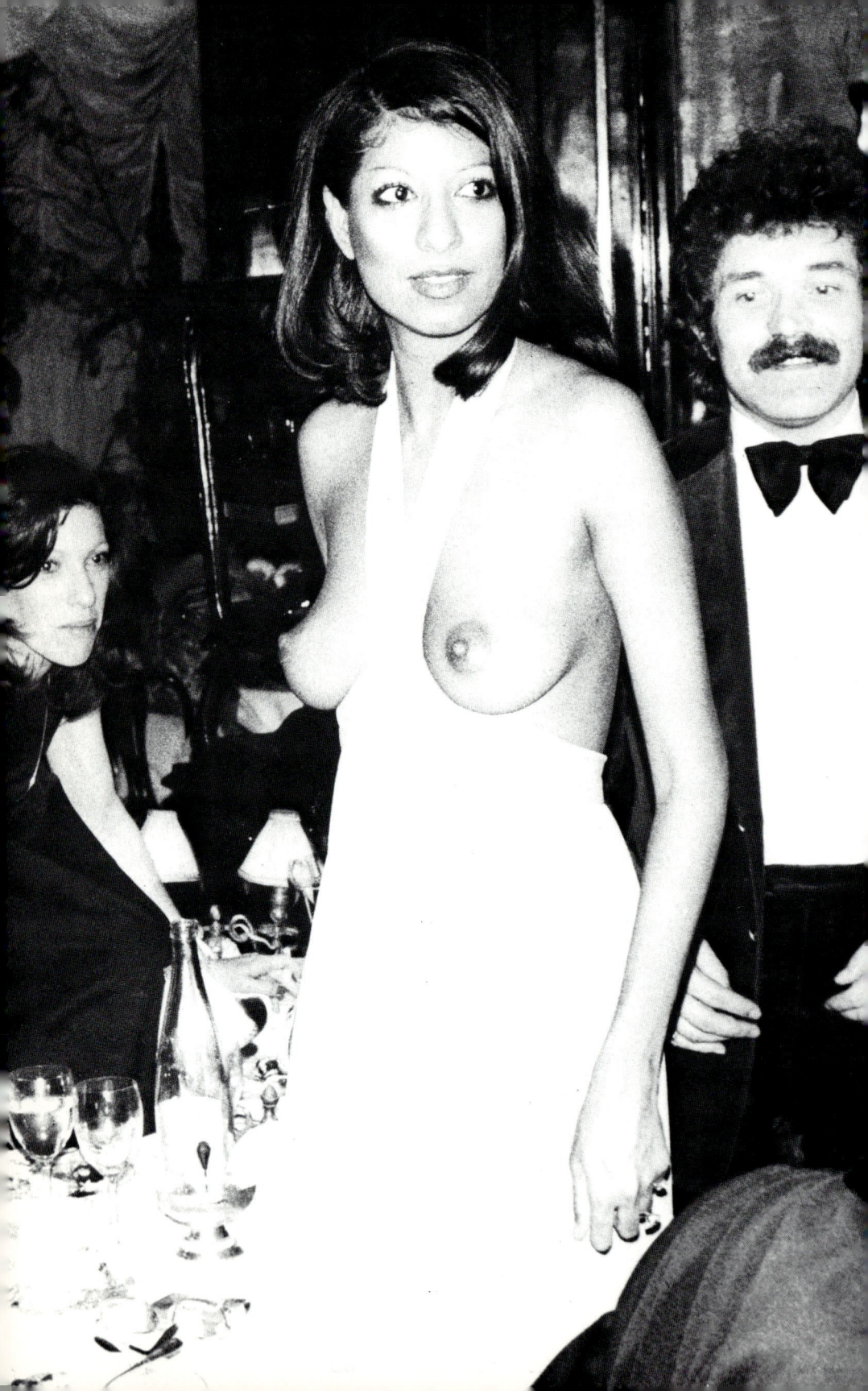

correspondingly rise and fall; thus, in the unending quest to secure male attention, interest is cunningly switched from site to site. In his study of modern American mores, *The Kandy Kolored Tangerine Flake Streamline Baby*, the journalist Tom Wolfe uncovered a tendency towards what he called 'buttocks décolletage'. The bustle was obviously another technique for directing attention to this part. The astonishing cod-pieces of the Renaissance were a male equivalent of this erotic attention-seeking.

Clothing has by now become far more than decoration, protection, seduction, or a device to ensure genital concealment. It has become a map of the face of a given culture. In this, it is similar to, but vastly more complex than, the body modification of primitives. In one's own country, one can enter a crowded room and discern a great deal about the social interrelations of those present from clothing and decoration. Nancy Mitford declared some years ago that the advent of cheap manufactured clothing had left only speech indicators to disclose rank. This is far from true. Hundreds of subtle indications as to social status are provided by clothing and ornament. If our society could be suddenly stripped naked, without having its modesty offended, chaos would undoubtedly supervene for a time since all the interactions between man and man as well as between man and woman would be deprived of their normal guide-lines. A complex civilization has an enormous investment in differentiated apparel. It is no accident that one of the first matters that a revolutionary regime turns its attention to is clothing. The French Revolution decreed classical grace and simplicity. The Chinese homogenized clothing. The Ayatollah Khomeini in Iran returned women to the black chador and so on.

Freud said that damming up the sexual impulse provided the energy for developing civilization. If this is true, the clutch of the machine is clothing. It is a regulator of enormous subtlety. It can switch in and switch out sexuality according to occasion and need. More, clothing can direct sexuality into productive channels and modulate it through various forms, including perverse ones, according to need. The essential condition for the harnessing of erotic energy for extra-erotic goals is genital concealment, and this is why all civilized clothing, no matter how provocative or suggestive it may be, demands such concealment. This fact is sensed, even if not admitted, by everyone with a vested interest in furthering one or another of the multifarious aims of civilization. Priests and politicians, educationalists and parents, lawyers and doctors, and the hydra-headed man and woman in the street all sense that the great machine of civilization can only be propelled onwards at the expense of free genital sexuality. Adam and Eve's aprons had embroidered on them a plan to conquer the universe.

The trouble is, the genitals will not lie down. As Flügel contends, they impudently emerge in symbolic form in the very instruments for their concealment, clothing. Much more hazardous to our future as conquerors of the cosmos is the fact that our genitals persistently manifest themselves in the technology we are forging for that conquest. Our titanic weaponry is, of course, almost unadulteratedly phallic. Many of our concepts of luxury, from armchairs to saloon cars, are womb fantasies. The bodily imagery can be extended. Our increasingly automated factories are metaphors for the body itself, devouring the earth and excreting consumer products. Our electronics and communications systems are, as McLuhan suggested, a global exteriorized nervous system. Where are the female genitals? Much less conspicuous, perhaps, because more heavily camouflaged. But in all service industries, public relations, the theatre and other entertainment, health, and money-manipulating concerns generally there is surely a flavour of them. Wherever people are wooed and seduced with promise of delight and increase or succour, there is the shadow of Eve's apron. Our peril, however, derives from the phallus substitutes, the great erect rockets with their inbuilt, cosmic orgasms. The concealing apron, so far from taming the penis, has produced a monstrous distortion in its rôle in the natural world. It is conceivable that if (*pace* Freud) we had been able to develop a technological culture without genital concealment it would display quite different and infinitely less perilous contours.

Corinna, in Swift's ironic poem 'A Beautiful Young Nymph Going to Bed' returns to her lodgings in the evening and:

> Pulls out the Rags contriv'd to prop
> Her flabby Dugs and down they drop.
> Proceeding on, the lovely Goddess
> Unlaces next her Steel-Rib'd Bodice;
> Which by the Operator's Skill,
> Press down the Lumps, the Hollows fill,
> Up goes her Hand, and off she slips
> The Bolsters that supply her Hips.
> With gentlest Touch, she next explores
> Her Shankers, Issues, running Sores . . .

Swift, in the poem, objectifies the vileness, 'shankers [i.e. venereal boils], issues [discharges], running sores', but there is abundant evidence elsewhere in Swift's work that the body itself, even in its healthy state, was for him a loathesome thing. He could never reconcile himself to physiological process. The unexpergated *Gulliver's Travels* is full of lamentation about excretion. Gulliver, in Brobdingnag, surveys the horrors of the giant maiden's body with disgust.

Swift was a highly civilized man. The eighteenth century in England, the Augustan age, is generally regarded, by upper-class Englishmen anyway, as one of the high-water marks of global civilization. Its taste in art, architecture, and literature, was flawless. Its speculative science and philosophy was ordered and progressive. Its education was classical and thorough, its life-style elegant. True, its satire and humour could be very earthy. The cartoons of Rowlandson and paintings of Hogarth are not squeamish. But it is significant that the intrusions of the licentious, raw body into this ordered and disciplined paradise was almost always satirical or pejorative. It did not harmonize properly with the Chippendale furniture, the Adam architecture or the artificial, if superb, landscapes of Capability Brown. It was felt nakedly by Swift, and doubtless less clearly by most, as a mutinous, buried threat to Civilization.

More than a century after Swift's death, another highly civilized man in another highly civilized place, Sigmund Freud in Vienna, published his influential theory of the structure of the human mind. He divided it into three constituents: the id, the ego and the super-ego. Put very briefly, the id is the instinctive, libidinous, pleasure-seeking part of the mind which exists beneath consciousness, the ego is the developed, self-conscious personality and the super-ego is the inbuilt authority which dictates individual and group morality. The id, throughout Freud's writing, is conceived of as dangerous, unpredictable, savage – a chained force in the basement of the mind sending up howls of despair and clamouring for release. Now the super-ego and the ego seem to be valid symbols of the structure of the human mind wherever it is found. The most primitive cultures have rules of conduct, standards of right and wrong, which are interiorized in each individual. But would any psychoanalyst be able to detect an id in an Australian aboriginal, a Kayapo Indian, a Nuer warrior or maiden? It is most unlikely. The id is, in fact, the projection of the body into the mind. It only emerges as a separate entity among people who have banished the body and its functions, especially unrestrained sexuality, from the fabric of their lives. People who live in and with their bodies do not have ids as civilized people do. Freud conceived the id as a danger to civilization but perhaps it is its imprisonment – the denial of the body – which is the real danger.

In an excellent science-fiction film, *The Forbidden Planet*, which was structured like Shakespeare's *The Tempest*, earth travellers find on a remote world the ruins of a civilization which has mysteriously perished after having constructed prodigies of sheer technology. The earthmen discover that the Krell, the vanished race, had developed a means to materialize their every thought. But they had forgotten, in their ancient wisdom and total civilization, the id. Their machines had begun to materialize 'monsters from the id' which ultimately destroyed them.

Our technology has a long way to go before it can equal such marvels, but it is moving fast. From balloons to space-ships in a century is no mean achievement, and there is reason to think that the development of technology obeys an exponential curve and is going to accelerate still more in the near future. We may not be able to objectify monsters from the id, but the rockets in their silos are perhaps a warning that we should set about making friends with our bodies again before it is too late.

THE FIG LEAF

> When we look back at this unashamed period of childhood it seems to us a Paradise; and Paradise itself is no more than a group phantasy of the childhood of the individual. That is why mankind were naked in Paradise and were without shame in one another's presence; till a moment arrived when shame and anxiety awoke, expulsion followed, and sexual life and the tasks of cultural activity began.

Probably only the final sentence-clause 'the tasks of cultural activity began' suggests the author of this, for him, surprisingly lyrical passage. It is Sigmund Freud. In fact, of course, there never was 'a moment' when 'shame and anxiety awoke'. The adoption by mankind of concealing clothing has been piecemeal and has proceeded at different rates in different parts of the world. Now that global civilization is effectively Western civilization, the wearing of concealing clothing is well-nigh universal, at least in cities. The genitals have been banished from the social scene.

Christianity was undoubtedly one of the chief instruments of their dismissal. Both the Old Testament and the New Testament are essentially hostile to sexuality and the body. It is true that there are passages in the Old Testament, such as Solomon's 'Song of Songs', which celebrate erotic passion. And when David, in a frenzy of rejoicing, danced almost naked before the Lord, and Saul's daughter rebuked him, it was she, and not David, who suffered as a result. For her small-minded abusiveness, she was made barren for life. But such episodes are rare. Generally speaking, the body was portrayed as something to be ashamed of. In *Leviticus*, the Lord tells Moses to convey to his people a series of sexual taboos. These begin: 'You shall not uncover the nakedness of your father, which is the nakedness of your mother; she is your mother, you shall not uncover her nakedness.' The Lord then gives a long list of what are essentially incest taboos, followed by various other prohibitions, including: 'You shall not lie with a male as with a woman; it is an abomination. And you shall not lie with any beast and defile yourself with it ... it is perversion.' Thus, with the formal interdiction of homosexuality and bestiality, this ancient text adumbrates the sexual morality which, enshrined in custom and law, has basically dominated Western civilization ever since the establishment of Christianity. Now incest taboos, and sexual prohibitions of different kinds, were certainly not confined to the ancient Hebrews. But because the Bible, as a result of its magnificent, sonorous prose, acquired a unique position as the chief sacred book of the world, its effect has been enormous.

The New Testament might have ameliorated the severity of the ancient Hebrew sexual taboos had it not been for the character of its chief apostle, Paul. He was a native of Tarsus where all the women were covered and veiled from head to foot and it might be said that through the vehemence with which he fulminated against unlawful sex and immodesty he managed to extend the borders of Tarsus to encompass the whole globe.

The development of the Pauline taboo is discussed by George Scott in *The Common Sense of Nudism*:

> Starting with the protection from public gaze of the sexual apparatus, it gradually extended its scope as the Christian Fathers hammered home their dictum that any part of the human body which was graceful or beautiful in curve or outline served to arouse passion in those who chanced to see it.

Certainly classical civilization had no horror of the body. The Greeks and the Romans were normally clothed but had no inhibitions about nakedness on special occasions. Athenaeus commended, as a delightful spectacle, young girls and men walking naked. St Chrysostom spoke of Roman women appearing nude in public, especially at the theatres, without shame or embarrassment. Plato recommended naked exercises for both sexes. Girls danced naked at Spartan feasts. Hippocrates, the father of medicine, recommended nude exposure to the sun as a cure as far back as 400 BC.

Although different cultures, under the aegis of different religious beliefs, have differed in their attitudes to the body, in Christianity is epitomized the doctrinal abhorrence of the body, as in pronouncements such as the following by Odon of Cluny: 'If men saw what is under the skin, endowed like the Boetian lynx with power to see within, the very sight of a woman would nauseate him.' Perhaps even more absurd is Gladstone's reaction to the passage in *The Odyssey* where Nausicaa and her maidens bathe the naked Odysseus:

> It is almost of itself incredible that habitually among persons of the highest rank and character, and without any necessity at all, such things should take place, and as it is not credible, so neither, I think, is it true.

By the time of Gladstone, and in the class of society to which he belonged, the body had vanished almost completely. It was not uncommon in Victorian England for people to spend their entire lives without ever seeing the naked human body and, in the case of certain exceptionally repressed people, especially women, this could include their own. Since then, of course, the grip of Christianity, at least in terms of sexual morality, has slackened considerably. Manners and customs have changed, and the body has made something of a comeback.

Among habitually naked peoples the body is secular and neutral. It is neither good nor bad. It is part of the environment like the ground, the sky, plants and animals. But once it has been banished a great many changes occur. The body is no longer morally neutral. This does not mean that it necessarily becomes evil. True, this has usually been its fate in Christian societies as the following passage from Jacques Boileau, writing in the seventeenth century, expresses very well:

> God hates nakedness, because he is purity itself; the Devil loves it, because he is impure: God hates nakedness, because it is a sign of our defeat and overthrow; and the Devil loves it, because it is a mark of his Triumph . . .

But is may also become the symbol of innocence and purity. At the height of Victorian repressiveness, Charles Kingsley, best known as the author of *The Water Babies*, who was also an Anglican divine, developed a private cult of nakedness. He practised private nudity and exhorted his future wife to do the same. Once the couple were married they maintained the tradition. In an early letter he wrote to her: 'When I feel very near God I always feel such a need to *undress*, as if everything which was artificial jarred me. What bliss to see that you feel the same.'

Kingsley also celebrated their mystical cult of nudity with a series of drawings which scandalized the few contemporaries privileged to see them.

A century earlier William Blake proclaimed that the nakedness of woman was the work of God, and tried to give practical expression to his belief by inviting his maid-servant to join him and his wife in nude sun-bathing. Mrs Blake, however, seems to have felt that the nakedness of woman was best taken in individual doses, and she vetoed the scheme.

The ambiguous status of the body in fact penetrated Christianity itself. While Christian theologians have, in general, always advocated, often to the point of obsession, modesty and concealment, the tradition of innocence associated with the *Genesis* story of Adam and Eve has always opened a door to the re-emergence of the body. Thus while it was common for girls raised in convents to be compelled to wear gowns while bathing, lest the sight of their own bodies inflame them and distress their heavenly protectors, some Christian sects adopted a defiant nakedness to stress their true, fundamentalist purity. The most recent of these has been the Doukhobors, originally a Russian group founded in the first half of the eighteenth century. Because they were pacifists, and rejected all external authority, the Doukhobors were in more or less continual conflict with the authorities. After being shunted around Russia for a century, seven thousand of them emigrated to Canada in 1899 in the hope of finding freedom to live in their own way. But the Canadian authorities kept trying to educate their children and extract taxes from the Doukhobors. The Doukhobors retaliated by marching naked on those they considered to be their persecutors. Large numbers were arrested. The naked marches have continued until quite recently although it seems the Doukhobors are slowly being assimilated into Canadian life.

In the fifteenth century, the Picards in Flanders worshipped naked and revered the body and before them, the Adamites in Bohemia, considered heretics and exterminated by John Zizka in 1421, not only went about naked to symbolize the innocence of Adam but practised free love in order to liberate the flesh. They taught that nakedness was essential to real purity and to the restoration of the innocence that had existed before the Fall. Men and women lived together in promiscuous groups. Their suppression was partly the result of claims by more orthodox Christians that the Adamites killed and terrorized those who refused to join them, but such claims are more often the result of envy than of truth.

It is common among primitive peoples to regard the genitals as powerful charms and sometimes as divinities. This is quite natural since the male and female sexual organs are the instruments for the propagation of life. Thus representations of the genitals were often worshipped or used as charms to protect people, animals and crops. Growing orchards might be inscribed with stylized representations of the vagina to ensure fruitfulness.

There are innumerable rites, both Christian and pagan, that involve nudity. The alleviation of barrenness in women is often magically helped by nakedness. Thus, in India, a barren woman, in order to make herself fertile, had to remove all her clothes and circle a fig tree 108 times, wrapping it round with a cotton thread. There is, of course, obvious sexual symbolism in this. The fig is, because of its colour and appearance, a common symbol of the female genitals. The Indian woman was thus wrapping the phallic trunk of the tree in a symbolic vagina, encouraged by the vaginal fruits which also symbolized the desired offspring.

In East Prussia, women sowed peas naked, in order to stimulate the vine to produce an abundance of the phallic fruit. In the Philippines, among the members of the Tagalog tribe, when a woman was in labour, it was the duty of her husband to climb onto the roof naked and brandish a sword and shield at the sky. In the meantime, naked friends below staged a mock fight. The purpose of this performance was to distract and frighten any evil spirits that might be lurking about in order to harm the mother and child.

Malignant spirits were by no means banished from the world with the advent of Christianity. The middle ages were much plagued by them. Two of the most notable were the incubus and the succubus, the former a devil in the guise of a man and the latter a devil in the guise of a woman. At night, while unsuspecting Christians slept, they might be visited by incubi and succubi who would copulate with them in their sleep. Now the danger of this was obviously considerably greater for women than for men since the women might find themselves bearing demonic offspring. In fact, the danger of impregnation by evil spirits has always haunted the consciousness of mankind and the genital leaf or apron, in addition to being a sexual lure or instrument of modesty (the two usually fusing ambivalently) was also considered a barrier to diabolic impregnation. But devils are cunning and can enter the body in many ways. St Paul, although a subtle theologian, was also a man of his times. He insisted on women covering their heads to prevent devils penetrating them through their ears. This custom is, of course, preserved in contemporary Christian worship but few women, donning their best hats for Sunday morning service, realize that they are doing so to avoid diabolic impregnation.

The Jews have always been in the forefront of the struggle against the body. Seymour Fisher, in his excellent *Body Consciousness* quotes a present-day Hasidic Jew defending his black, large-brimmed hat, long black coat and white knee socks:

> With my appearance I cannot attend a theatre or movie or any other places where a religious Jew is not supposed to go. Thus, my beard and my sidelocks and my Hasidic clothing serve as a guard and a shield from sin and obscenity.

In Mark's Gospel, after Judas has kissed Jesus and thus delivered him to his enemies, Jesus is led away to judgement, crucifixion and the dawn of Christianity. All desert him except for a mysterious young man who 'followed him, with nothing but a linen cloth about his body; and they seized him, but he left the linen cloth and ran away naked.' It is tempting to see in that anonymous youth, who makes such a fleeting appearance in history, a symbol of the body fleeing the dispensation to come.

In modern Western society there are few survivals of body magic. True, every public toilet contains obscene drawings and often stylized representations of, usually male, genitals. These doubtless contain some residual magical charge but they are much closer to pornography. Anyone who has read Freud knows that church-steeples, maypoles and so on are phallic symbols. So, of course, is a skyscraper or indeed a telegraph pole but by now utility has probably drained such objects of magical potency. The revolver in Western movies is a true phallic symbol, epitomizing a large part of the cultural ideal of masculinity in the West, which is distressingly rooted in machismo and death-dealing.

Once concealed, the body can become a symbol of both evil and innocence and also in itself a kind of magical charm or amulet. In May, 1979, Emperor Bokassa, in reality a minor Central African tyrant, arrested a large number of children on charges of sedition and massacred some of them. According to *The Guardian* (London) of 18 May, 'Hundreds of women demonstrated naked outside the prison until the survivors were released.' These women were not consciously employing magic to procure the release of their children but they were making use of the age-old coercive power of the naked body.

'Concealment' does not, in fact, invariably mean genital concealment. Shame can attach itself to very varied parts of the body. The mouth and oral cavity is often the recipient and there are people who will excrete, or even copulate, publicly but will never eat in public. It has been said that if a woman were surprised in her bath, she would cover, if she were a Moslem her face, if a Chinese her feet, if a Sumatran her knees, if a Samoan her navel, if a Laotian her breasts and if she were an Alaskan she would put the ornamental plug back in her lip. But the overwhelming majority of women, as well as men, would cover the genital parts. Shame may, in certain cases, have migrated to improbable sites but its true home, in concealed cultures, is the genitals.

It is interesting to speculate as to what kind of model of the human mind Sigmund Freud would have constructed if he had based it not on clothed Europeans but on, say, a study of the naked Nuer of the Sudan. Almost all the processes which he discerns as formative for the adult mind would have been lacking. Freud assumes that children will not normally see each other naked and that, if they do happen to, the result will be traumatic. This is not true of naked cultures. He assumes that sexual play and masturbation will be ruthlessly suppressed and punished. Again, this is not true of naked cultures. Thus great provinces of Freud's mind-empire would simply be missing. There would be no Oedipus complex (or not much, anyway), no penis envy or castration complex, probably no clear-cut phases of sexual development. We are emerging rapidly from the era of Freudian gospel, while retaining respect for the Viennese doctor as a true originator, and can now perceive the extent to which he himself was the victim of prevailing ideas and prejudices. The womens' liberation movement indignantly refuted much of elementary Freudianism and indeed such analyses of his as the following, concerning penis envy, now seem bizarre indeed:

> After a woman has become aware of the wound to her narcissism, she develops, like a scar, a sense of inferiority. When she has passed beyond her first attempt at explaining her lack of penis as being a punishment personal to herself and has realized that that sexual character is a universal one, she begins to share the contempt felt by men for a sex which is the lesser in so important a respect . . .

Freud lived in the age of the supremacy of mechanical engineering. His models of the mind are very similar to engineer's constructs, and indeed, the assembled super-ego, ego and id can be compared to a steam locomotive. The steam is the id (generated by the fires of hell), which, suitably repressed, propels the ego-locomotive along the tracks, the whole powerful, rackety structure precariously controlled by the super-ego-driver. The parts may be of different construction and efficiency but they are essentially immutable. It seems increasingly evident that the mind is far more protean than Freud suspected and that it can change the fundamental character of its individual parts and overall appearance. The engineering model is invalid.

Nevertheless, the transition from an animal state to that of fully-concealed civilized man can be meaningfully related to broad changes in sexual behaviour. Let us briefly examine this evolution, starting with a look at the higher primates.

The following observations were made by Zuckerman in the London zoo. The first concerns a six-month-old, pig-tailed monkey and its mother:

> During its explorations of its mother's body, and often in the midst of play-fighting activities, it would suddenly stop and peer at her pudendal region ... When it was about six months old, it mounted its mother in response to her repeated presentation, and about a month later this activity was first seen to be accompanied by erection and by pelvic thrusts. About this stage it was often observed presenting both to its mother and to neighbouring animals. Sometimes, when it mounted her, its mother pulled it off; at other times she seemed to incite it to cover her ...

The next concerns young male baboons:

> They employ sexual approach in obtaining access to each other and to entice a fellow for play. They masturbate and they mount each other. They mount and are mounted by adult males and by adult females ... They engage in manual, oral and olfactory ano-genital examination with animals of their own age and with adults of both sexes.

Clearly, there are no inhibitions, no rules or conventions governing erotic activity which is simply a constituent of the flow of experience. Probably the only aspect of (some) primate, as well as other mammalian, sexual behaviour which has any significance for the later development of human sexual morality is the harem-building impulse which motivates the old males to assemble a private harem of nubile females, driving the younger and weaker males out of the group where they may be forced into unwilling celibacy. This kind of behaviour is, of course, much more conspicuous in the wild than in zoos.

Incidentally, all primates do not form either harems or 'pair-bonds'. Chimpanzees, for example, live an essentially promiscuous group life although dominant males tend to monopolize females.

Writing in 1918, Freud remarked: 'Many observers of primitive races living today have put forward the view that their impulsions in love are relatively weak and never reach the degree of intensity which we are accustomed to meet with in civilized men.' In the sense that a dammed river builds up more pressure than a freely flowing one, this is undoubtedly true. Perhaps the chief distinction between primitive and civilized attitudes to sex is that, in primitive cultures, childhood sexuality is usually tolerated. Whatever the degree of adult suppression of free-flowing eroticism, and this may be severe, children are usually allowed, or even encouraged, to masturbate and engage in erotic play. This contrasts sharply with what, until very recently, has been the attitude of civilization to childhood sexuality. Freud, at the turn of the century, takes it for granted that masturbation will be punitively suppressed and it is safe to say that throughout the Christian era in the West childhood sexuality has been at the very least actively discouraged. But it is in childhood that ineradicable attitudes are formed which will condition an individual's responses throughout his life. In primitive societies, each individual usually has some experience of Eden. In civilized ones, he or she is virtually born outside the walls.

The world of clothed fellow beings is a strange one. The object of one of the most powerful instinctual drives is both omnipresent and invisible. This object is, of course, the genitals of the opposite sex. Every individual is perpetually conscious of sexual allure radiating from the concealed parts that, under normal conditions, surround him or, of course, her, and of being stringently prohibited from following the dictates of instinct. Most of the behaviour of primates described above has now become forbidden to man. It is either actually illegal or classified as perversion or, at the least, deprecated. There is voyeurism, various kinds of incest, homosexuality, indecent assault, exhibitionism, *de facto* rape and so on. Through this enchanted wood of erotic play, civilization has hacked out a narrow trail which represents all that remains lawful. Basically, this permitted path, although it has perhaps ramified a little in recent decades, consists of a little premarital 'petting' followed by life-long monogamy. But although it is possible for human beings to walk this path, it is quite impossible for them to do so naturally and fulfillingly. Hence our culture is perfused with escaping eroticism. It is astonishing how, in the late nineteenth century, perversions multiplied. So narrow did the permitted trail for the passage of the instincts become that a great and humane writer like Tolstoy could take the absurd position of maintaining that *all* sexual contact was wicked and it would be better, even at the expense of the survival of the human race, if it were abolished. Poor Tolstoy was obviously fighting a titanic battle against his own healthy and vigorous sexual instincts.

When the naked Nuer girls prepare for a night-long dance, which will end, for most of them, in love-making, they *put on* leather skirts. The skirt, concealing clothing, intensifies male desire. This is why civilized people have such hair-trigger erotic responses. Freud basically regarded humour as an explosive discharge of neural energy. Analysing obscene and sexual humour, he remarks: 'A chance exposure had a comic effect on us because we compare the ease with which we have enjoyed the sight with the great expenditure which would otherwise be required for reaching this end.' If Freud was right in supposing that instinctual repression is essential for building a high civilization then New York and London are constructed quite as much of clothes as of bricks and mortar. It is no wonder that Norman O. Brown in his profound work *Life Against Death* ultimately concluded that a city is 'crystallized guilt'.

Through the city of 'crystallized guilt', clothed man weaves an endless dance of frustrated eroticism. The preliminaries and accessories of sexuality are substituted for the essence. Punctuated it is true by some genital contact, lawful or adulterous, moderns essentially flirt endlessly, ogle, circle, skirt, brush, skirmish but rarely unite.

In *Deuteronomy* 22.5, Moses proclaimed that 'A woman shall not wear anything that pertains to a man, nor shall a man put on a woman's garment; for whosoever does these things is an abomination to the Lord your God.' Two thousand years later in *The Anatomie of Abuse*, written in 1583, Philip Stubbes insisted 'Our apparell was given as a signe distinctive to discerne betwixt sex and sex; and therefore, one to wear the apparell of another sexe is to participate with the same, and to adulterate the veritie of his own kinde.'

But what, exactly, is 'the veritie of his own kinde'? With the passing ages it has become less and less clear. Clothes have certainly proved inadequate designators of gender. It is perhaps true to say that, in the broadest sense, form-fitting lower garments characterize the male sex and the open dress the female but there are so many exceptions, which include whole civilizations (the Roman toga and the Japanese kimona were both unisex), as to make the pronouncement of small classificatory value. There are abundant examples of garments which, in one culture, would have been considered masculine and in another feminine. Much more important, psychologically, is the consideration that there are always individuals who identify with the opposite sex and strive to wear its clothes.

Gender is a more superficial thing that it is generally supposed. Every human being's mind contains feminine and masculine components and every human being's body contains male and female hormones. Undoubtedly there are real sexual differences, related to reproductive function, physical strength and profile, cerebral and neural subtleties, but the common image, which has required repeated shoring up by theologians like Moses and others with a cultural interest in maintaining the rigid distinction, of male and female as virtually different species, is untenable. Throughout nature, the female is the archetype of the species and the male is essentially a fertilizing machine which, in the case of some very primitive species, is not even necessary, as the females reproduce parthenogenetically, without the intervention of fertilizing males. In human beings too, the female is the archetype and the male, who retains vestigial female breasts, is an adaptation for fertilizing purposes. Almost certainly, if there were no cultural pressures of any kind, men and women would be much closer to each other in thought and behaviour. There are some who see in the recognition of our essential bisexuality, a path towards a new Eden. Dr Charlotte Wolff, a psychiatrist, maintains that 'Human sexuality and love has been crippled, falsified, suppressed. But there is beginning a new richness, through the recognition that we are all both male and female . . .'

Undoubtedly, it is not as simple as that. There have been innumerable sexual false dawns before and will be again. No matter how attractive sweeping solutions may seem, history invariably shows them to have been simplistic. The partial ambiguity of human gender is itself responsible. In ages where feminine impulses dominate, the masculine consciousness musters its machismo for a counter attack. And vice versa. There is always tomorrow and the possibility of new trends and what is possible will be explored by mankind. Two beings were driven out of Eden, Adam and Eve, and they, clad in the concealing aprons which magnify and distort their erotic instinct, will have to pursue their uneasy coexistence through many novel alignments for a long time to come.

THE NUDE

So far, this book has been concerned chiefly with living people and the next chapter will return to them. But this chapter will examine images of the body and their significance for human culture as well as their interaction, sometimes a very direct one, with living people. There can hardly be a better starting point than a quotation from one of the most eminent, and perceptive, living men to have concerned himself deeply with art and, especially, with 'The Nude'. The following quotation does not, however, come from Lord Clark's celebrated book of that title but consists of a brief statement he made to Lord Longford's committee investigating pornography. It is fairly long but because it defines the area to be covered by this chapter, and mentions most of the specific subjects, it deserves quoting in full:

> To my mind art exists in the realm of contemplation and is bound by some sort of imaginative transposition. The moment art becomes an incentive to action it loses its true character. This is my objection to painting with a communist programme, and it would also apply to pornography. In a picture like Correggio's *Danae* the sexual feelings have been transformed, and although we undoubtedly enjoy it all the more because of its sensuality, we are still in the realm of contemplation. The pornographic wall-paintings in Pompeii are documentaries and have nothing to do with art. There are one or two doubtful cases – a small picture of copulation by Gericault and a Rodin bronze of the same subject. Although each of these is a true work of art, I personally feel that the subject comes between me and complete aesthetic enjoyment. It is like too strong a flavour added to a dish. There remains the extraordinary example of Rembrandt's etching of a couple on a

bed, where I do not find the subject at all disturbing because it is seen entirely in human terms and is not intended to promote action. But it is, I believe, unique, and only Rembrandt could have done it.*

Up to now in this book I have used the word 'nude' as roughly synonymous with 'naked'. No apology is needed. The Oxford Dictionary ratifies this use, defining the word, when applied to the human figure, as meaning 'Naked, undraped'. The arbitrary imposition of jargon terminology is deprecable and, in general, words should be left as flexible as possible. There are, however, good grounds for making a distinction between 'naked' and 'nude'. Lord Clark begins his study of undraped figure painting and sculpture, *The Nude*, with the following distinction:

> The English language, with its elaborate generosity, distinguishes between the naked and the nude. To be naked is to be deprived of our clothes and the word implies some of the embarrassment which most of us feel in that condition. The word nude, on the other hand, carries, in educated usage, no uncomfortable overtone. The vague image it projects into the mind is not of a huddled and defenceless body, but of a balanced, prosperous and confident body: the body re-formed.

There is, in fact, no philological justification for Lord Clark's proposed distinction. Both words stem, by different roots, from the old Sanskrit 'nagnag' which had an in-built connotation of shame. It does, however, reflect a real need that has been increasingly felt by art critics and historians to discriminate between a certain kind of stylized and usually idealized representation of the body and a merely naked body. One might say that the model in an art class is naked, the drawings that the students are making from him or her are nude, although one might have to add that the pose, formality and above all situation of the model means that he or she acquires some of the properties of the nude.

Two-dimensional and three-dimensional images (paintings and sculpture) of naked bodies of one kind or another have been produced in all parts of the world and back to remote paleolithic times, 20,000 and more years ago. Lord Clark maintains that 'the nude' was 'an art form invented by the Greeks in the 5th century BC', but this is a

*Pornography – The Longford Report: copyright © 1972, by the members of the Longford Committee Investigating Pornography. First published by Coronet Books, 1972. Reprinted by permission of Hodder and Stoughton Limited.

somewhat arbitrary ascription. What Lord Clark is clearly referring to is 'prosperous' and relatively naturalistic images in the Western tradition. The distinction he makes between 'naked' and 'nude' images is taken up by another eminent modern critic of very different cultural orientation, the Marxist, John Berger. He or one of his collaborators writes in *Ways of Seeing*:

> In his book on *The Nude*, Kenneth Clark maintains that to be naked is simply to be without clothes, whereas the nude is a form of art. According to him, a nude is not the starting point of a painting, but a way of seeing which the painting achieves. To some degree, this is true ... A naked body has to be seen as an object in order to become a nude ... The nude is condemned to never being naked. Nudity is a form of dress.

The paradox is valid. There is a great gulf, in the classical European tradition, between a naked body and 'a nude'. This expresses itself in many ways. There is, almost invariably, a sense in the nude of pose. This, of course, is partly because the models actually were posed but in many cases the artists thought that they were posing them in life-like ways. Yet invariably there is a sense of the unnatural rather than of frozen motion. Among many subjects which have given European painters an excuse to paint nude female bodies is the rape of the Sabine women by the Romans. Naked and partially-clad women are usually scattered about the canvas. Horsemen scoop up lamenting damsels. Everywhere there is struggle and confusion – but no real movement! The scene is 'composed'. It is hypostasized. It has no conceivable moment before or moment after. Everyone in the picture has adopted a *pose plastique*. The very essence of life, which is motion, is not only not shown, which a still picture naturally cannot do, nor even suggested, but has been formally proscribed. It is worth recalling that in Victorian music halls, and even into the 1950s in burlesque shows like the one at the Windmill Theatre in London, girls were allowed to appear 'undraped' on stage as long as they did not move. They were also usually posed unnaturally. Robbed of motion they were also purged of the offence of being naked. They became 'nudes'.

There are many other things which distinguish a nude in a painting or sculpture from a naked man or woman. The nude is usually placed in an idealized setting, classic or pastoral, bears unnatural wisps of clothing or adornment, is of unlikely physical perfection and has atrophied genitals.

The nude, from early Renaissance times until quite recently, was regarded as the zenith of art. Landscape, still life, genre painting, decorative art, early surrealism, and many other forms flourished but the nude was treated with almost religious reverence. The stature of an artist was judged by his handling of the nude. Women were strictly barred from that chapel of aesthetic religion, the life-class. Clarence Norwood, an advocate of nudism writing in 1933, remarks: 'The study of the nude has always been regarded as a legitimate branch of plastic art. Why this should be so has never been convincingly explained.' There is indeed a considerable mystery here. Is it really so much more challenging to paint a man's body than a donkey's body, a female breast or limb than an oak tree or a bullrush, a male torso than a landscape? The answer is, of course, that it is not. The subject is more or less irrelevant as a test of the artist's skill. Whence then comes the mystique of 'the nude'? The clue can be found in another remark by Clarence Norwood: 'Seeing that the average member of the public has little or no chance of comparing the artistic product with reality . . .' Of course! That is what the European nude is an essence – the banished body! The body has been uprooted from nature and hung on the wall. There is a balancing mechanism in the mind which reasserts at least a semblance of sane values no matter what the psychotic fantasies imposed upon human beings by authority. As the body vanished under concealing clothing the impulse to regain it, if only in effigy, became more and more imperative and set the painters and sculptors of the world churning out replicas of it. But, in order not too provocatively to confront the ecclesiastical and other law-givers who had decreed its dismissal, the re-emergent image of the body was censored and sufficiently denatured to make it uneasily tolerated.

This is not, of course, the whole story. Nothing ever is, since all things ultimately form a continuum. But it is undoubtedly a very important and insufficiently recognized part of it. It is a striking fact that naked peoples do not produce naturalistic images of the human body. They may draw birds, animals, trees and plants with great skill and representational power, but the body is almost always distorted. There is no paradox. If one asks why they represent nature reasonably accurately but distort the body, the answer is that there are far more important things to be said about the body, and represented allegorically and symbolically in painting and sculpture, than its mere surface appearance. A bird or a tree may be magically distorted or it may be shown as it is. But, to people surrounded by naked human forms, there seems little point in reproducing them in wood, stone or pigment. What is important about the body is its fierceness, its frailty, its nobility, its fertility, its creativity and many other attributes which naturalistic paintings generally do not show. Therefore primitive representations of the body – which Picasso and others have rightly taught us to esteem if not always to understand – are almost invariably symbolic constructs which have a mythical or magical significance. It is only a concealed culture which can become obsessed with the surface appearance of people.

The natural next question is: what of the Greeks? True, they wore clothes but they were friends with their own bodies. There were abundant occasions for nakedness in Greek life. The Greeks painted and sculpted nude bodies, certainly, just as they painted and sculpted clothed ones. They painted and sculpted people naked and clothed and driving their cattle to market and getting drunk and making love and wrestling and running and – in virtually all the postures of life. The nude may have sprung from Greek roots but its monstrous overemphasis and detachment from an equally intense interest with the other aspects of lived life is essentially non-Greek. The posed, denatured nude of the European tradition would be alien to the dynamic Greek notion of art.

If the Greeks 'invented the nude' they also invented pornography. It is a nice question as to when representations of human beings copulating and indulging in every form of orgiastic excess change from being mystical celebrations of vitality and become 'filth'. Many people would consider explicit erotic scenes on Greek vases, Indian temples and possibly Japanese and Tantric drawings and paintings to be the former and identical photographed scenes sold under the counter in Soho and Times Square, and indeed almost everywhere, to be the latter. The psychology of this key ambivalence is worth examining.

'The moment' Lord Clark explained in the passage quoted above, 'art becomes an incentive to action it loses its true character.' As regards the consumer of art, according to this proposition, art must be inert. It must not disturb his, or her, exquisite equilibrium. It must not have 'too strong a flavour', causing the viewer to choke or splutter or make any bodily adjustments at all. This is, *par excellence*, art as seen by an upper-class European. In this context, one does not have to be a Marxist to see that John Berger's persistent critique of the relationship between Western art and the 'connoisseur' is correct. It is the relationship between merchandize and wealthy consumer. The world of art, like the world itself, is essentially an emporium through which the civilized man can browse and purchase, without having his psychological composure endangered. The 'nude' has 'no uncomfortable overtone'. The viewer is not compelled to take the appropriate action when coming upon a 'huddled and defenceless body' but can delight, safely and without action, in a 'balanced, prosperous and confident body'. But the dimension of action of primary concern here is not so much economic or cultural as sexual. For Lord Clark, before a work can be considered art, the sexual feelings must be 'transformed'. Otherwise it becomes 'disturbing'. What does he mean? He means it would produce a sexual response, generate the appropriate physical manifestation, which in a man would be an erection, and might even impel the viewer to 'action'. What action? Masturbation, most likely, or else, if the circumstances permitted, perhaps some kind of sexual intercourse with another person. But if a work did this then it could not possibly be art, but must be pornography. And, despite Indian temples and tantric prints, for Western aesthetes in general, the two are forever incompatible. A work cannot be both art and pornography. The maintenance of this unconvincing dogma inevitably creates the most appalling metaphysical contortions. Look at Lord Clark on Rembrandt's etching of copulation: 'I do not find the subject at all disturbing because it is seen entirely in human terms and is not intended to promote action.' In *human* terms? Is sexuality then essentially inhuman? What he probably means is that the couple represented are convincing, lifelike, naturalistic. But this surely makes the scene more, not less, erotic. Compare Rembrandt's etching with Guilio Romano's where the couples illustrating copulatory positions have all the vitality of lamp-posts. Which is the more erotic? Surely the Rembrandt and surely it is then more likely to 'promote action'. But still it is not *intended* to. Well, it is a wise historian who can assert that positively.

'The pornographic wall-paintings in Pompeii are documentaries and have nothing to do with art.' It is interesting that George Bernard Shaw, an exceptionally prudish man, attempted to detach James Joyce from the stigma of being a pornographer by calling *Ulysses* 'a document'. If something can be relegated to the category of 'document' then it can be safely dismissed from critical attention as art while being implicitly condoned for its seriousness of purpose. In fact, it appears most unreasonable to dismiss the Pompeian murals as documentaries. They are, in every respect, as much works of art as Masaccio's murals, as Indian temple sculptures or – as thousands upon thousand of works showing explicit sexual scenes.

A woman novelist once said that she was against pornography because it was 'the enemy of art'. There is surely only one interpretation that can be given such a remark, that the weed of pornography is so vigorous that it must be hacked down if the delicate flower of art is to live. This implies a miserably condescending attitude to art. If it is that feeble is it of any use to anyone? The truth, of course, is that no valid distinction whatsoever can be made between pornography and art because they are not comparable things. Pornography, rightly considered, is a constituent, and an important one, of art, not a rival cultural domain. There can be works of art which are devoid of pornography. There can be works of art which are little else but pornography. And there can, of course, be pornography which is not art at all, just as there can be works dealing with any branch of life which are not art. The impossible task that censors in all ages have set themselves is to separate pornographic art from non-artistic pornography. It is impossible because art always transcends the consciousness of its age and therefore no representatives of that consciousness can judge it. Great art, which, as in Shakespeare's plays, may include pornographic elements, transcends the consciousness of all the ages.

When the tenth-century Indian temples, bristling with erotic statuary, were first built, doubtless some Brahmins of the time fulminated at the outrage. Now they are seen as priceless cultural treasures. In every age, there have been those who have greeted explicit sexual representations, in print, stone or pigment, with pharisaic horror and have tried to mobilize opinion against them. In our day, it is photographs which are the chief victims of such assaults. And yet, is an orgy on the bottom of a Greek cup any less pornographic than an orgy on film? It may be that the shamefaced men shuffling into 'porn shops' in fact represent a healthier spirit than the self-appointed guardians of morality. In any case, the human race will not be divorced from the body and its functions. The struggle between the censors and the populace results in many strange and paradoxical confrontations and reversals. For example, Lord Clark's admirable study, *The Nude* was first published in 1956 when the body was much suppressed. Can he, or anyone else, seriously doubt that one reason for its enormous success was the, admittedly partially denatured, bodies it purveyed? Is Lord Clark a pornographer? Lord Longford probed long and superficially into the question of pornography. The monumental report on his tendentious researches was published in a paperback volume, bearing on the front, in enormous red letters occupying two-thirds of the available space PORNOGRAPHY. Chastely nestling below it is a circle with the qualifying words in small print, 'The Longford Report'. It was, as the publishers cannily realized, the eternal and essentially wholesome lure of the flesh which induced the public to purchase the assault on it.

Much of scholarly wisdom is only successfully imposed dogma. Art should not, according to Lord Clark, incite to action. According to Philip Rawson in his introduction to the Tantra Exhibition in London, in 1971:

> Hindu Tantra [cultivates] activities aimed especially at arousing the libido, dedicating it, and ensuring that the mind is not indulging in mere phantasy. All the concrete enjoyments and imagery are supposed to awaken dormant energies, especially the energy which normally finds its outlet in sexual intercourse. The energy, once aroused, is harnessed to rituals, meditation and yoga, turned back up within the human energy-mechanism, and used to propel the consciousness towards blissful enlightenment.

Lest this admittedly convoluted statement sound like a programme for 'sublimation' it should be said that the induced orgasm is a key element in the enlightenment attained. Here is a proposition diametrically opposed to Lord Clark's: the essential purpose of art is to induce action. True art can be both passive and active, soothing or an incitement to action, pornographic, non-pornographic, or a combination of these and other elements. True art does not consist solely in those works a civilized inheritor of the classical/Christian tradition would choose to house in his rooms or travel to view.

John Berger or one of his co-authors (each writes anonymously) remarks:

> In ... non-European traditions – in Indian art, Persian art, African art, Pre-columbian art – nakedness is never supine ... And if, in these traditions, the theme of a work is sexual attraction, it is likely to show active sexual love as between two people, the woman as active as the man, the actions of each absorbing the other.

There is, in fact, a peculiar isolation about the Western nude. Sometimes the subjects are named, and occasionally they are shown with lovers or other allegedly close relatives or associates, and yet these posed figures seem to represent beings insulated from biological reality. Individuals in clothed cultures are separated from what Margaret Mead called 'close bodily contact' with their peers and relatives. They are isolated in little cultural worlds: their clothing. Perhaps one strong constituent of the Western tradition of the nude is that it provides assurance that the body does still exist intact, healthy and unmutilated even though it has been detached from the flow of experience by clothing. European nudes are not naked people, but clothed people without their clothes.

Lawrence Langer notes that painters and sculptors of the Western nude tradition

> . . . usually find that the complete uncovering of the human body is embarrassing because it brings mankind's lower centers too prominently into view . . . *Conventional morality plays a part in this, but more important is the artist's wish to depict his subject without offending against mankind's desire for superiority over the animal world.* [his italics].

One's first thought is that a species lacking genitals or with shrivelled genitals has small claim to any such superiority. However, it is clear what Langer means. The nude shares with all Western art, produced in countries dominated by Christianity, an aspiration towards 'the spiritual'. Art, according to Lord Clark, 'exists in the realm of contemplation and is bound by some sort of imaginative transposition'. This is an attempt at a secular formulation of an essentially theological pronouncement. Christianity has always divided people up into physical and spiritual parts, of which the latter is incomparably the more fortunate and the nobler. The body is 'dust'. It decays. It is brutish and unredeemed, the heir to gross tides and impure aspirations. The spirit is immortal and immutable and will ultimately, if the wicked body hasn't prejudiced its chances too gravely, actually soar up to unite with the Creator of the Universe. All graphic art, to some extent, vibrates to this spirit of mystical transfiguration. A landscape is not merely a landscape, but a province of the divine. A bowl of fruit is testimony to the munificence and immanence of the Lord of Hosts. And a nude – is an angel in its caterpillar stage. In the works of Blake, for example, many of the nudes actually resemble human butterflies taking wing.

Once, however, the dichotomy between body and spirit has become accepted, it becomes a handy metaphor to project onto the body itself. Because, in Christian theology, the body is not uniformly depraved. The heart is noble, inheriting some of the prestige of the Sacred Heart of Christ. The 'mind' (not really a physical constituent at all) is receptive to noble and pious truths and can in its turn infuse the body with seemly conduct. The breast or bosom (again a symbolic rather than genuinely physical component) fills with pity which is holy, and so on. But, further down, there is little of virtue. In fact, the whole bodyscape below the belt is a sorry prospect. There is the seat of excretion – and does not the devil himself live at *anus mundi*? But, far worse, there is the seat of the passions, responsible for Adam and Eve's downfall, in some rather nebulous way. Many of the chief theological sins and vices have their roots in the genitals. The ano-genital complex is almost a map of hell. In Boccaccio's delightful story a naughty monk seduces an innocent girl by telling her that he has a devil attached to him and he can only be redeemed if it is put safely into hell which, fortunately, the girl is equipped with.

The American wit, H.L. Mencken had the ingenious idea of arranging the parts of the body into a hierarchy of eight classes starting with respectable ones and descending to those which, in 1915 when he was writing, were utterly unmentionable. Such analytical subtlety is unnecessary for the present purpose. It is enough to say that there has always been, in Western society, a sense that the upper part of the body is good and the lower part debased.

It is this theological aura of damnation which has cast a blight on the genitals of Western nudes. It is, of course, a fact much observed and pondered upon but little discussed that some grave affliction infects these parts. Women's abdomens often end in a featureless pink triangle. Men's reproductive parts, when posture, or convenient obstruction, does not eclipse them totally are usually shrunken and faded. There are, naturally, variations in intensity of genital display but it is probably true to say that, with very rare exceptions, the genitals of nudes are rarely comparable with their models in naked reality. What a contrast with the rest of the body in art! There, everything is 'prosperous'. Muscles are ripe and bulging, hair glossy and abundant, faces lovingly detailed and bold.

In truth, the genitals do provide a real dilemma to artists. Freud remarked sadly, 'We never regard the genitals themselves, which produce the strongest sexual excitation, as really "beautiful".' The genitals are, of course, intrinsically as 'beautiful' as an ear or a toe or any other constituent of the body but, as Freud aptly pointed out, they 'produce the strongest sexual excitation'. And it is that sexual excitation which provides a dilemma to painter or sculptor. If a nude is represented with all its parts, including genitals, in proportion to reality, the eye of the beholder, in a clothed society, will distort it. His or her eye will be drawn irresistibly to the genitals and they will grow out of all proportion to their physical prominence. It is quite probable that the atrophied genitals on Western nudes represent a kind of deliberate distortion, like that in architectural features designed to create a particular effect, in order to show a body that will be brought into ratio by the mind of the viewer.

In psychological truth, the genitals can never be shown in true proportion in works of art. They must be distorted. But there are two forms this distortion can take. The Western nude, under the aegis of Christianity, has shrunk them to produce the *illusion* of 'a balanced, prosperous and confident body: the body re-formed'. Or they can be exaggerated in order to make their appearance conform to their actual psychological significance. This is the method that is usually chosen by non-Western art. The genitals in Japanese erotic prints, Indian temple sculpture, Pompeian and other Roman murals and sculpture and most primitive sculpture are often represented as enormous, sometimes equivalent in size to the rest of the body. To the civilized eye, nourished on the Western nude, such representations seem grotesque and this effect is exploited by Aubrey Beardsley in some of his erotic works painted in England at the end of the last century. Beardsley is not painting the hypertrophied, symbolic genitals as seen by non-Christian artists, but a parody of them that represents the shock effect they have for the Western viewer. To the primitives and others who represent the human body with huge genitals there is no more sense of distortion than there is to the Westerners contemplating their nudes with atrophied genitals. There is symmetry and proportion. The genitals loom enormous in the conciousness, and that is the way the artists have represented them.

So significant, indeed, are the genitals to some pagan and primitive minds that they become detached from the body and may be painted or sculpted on their own. In psychological terms, a huge sculpted phallus is just as much a nude as a sculpted man with a fig-leaf over his genitals. The religion of the West deprecates the genitals and tries to dismiss them from its art and thought. But the religions of many other peoples exalt them. It is thus not at all unnatural for a woman to give up her virginity not to a man but an image of a god. Ritual defloration on a sculpted phallus has been practised in some parts of the world. Thus the work of art and lived reality fuse in a moment of biological significance.

There is an extremely secularized survival of this practice in the use of the masturbatory aid called the 'dildo', which has also been known as 'the little man'. A phallus of wood, rubber, plastic or some other substance has been used by women for erotic purposes since before language, if its use by chimpanzees can be taken as evidence. Such aids are, in fact, tiny, functional nudes. Nowadays, of course, they are often electrified and called 'vibrators'. In psychological terms, the vibrator and the classic Western male nude with atrophied genitals define the spectrum of Western sexuality.

If the 'prosperous' Western nude can sometimes functionally contract to a cylinder of electrified plastic it can also, thanks to modern plastic and prosthetic surgery, affect the body in another way. The nude can, as it were, become flesh and walk. There is no doubt that the idealized images of the Western nude tradition, which, in secular form but essentially unmodified, are carried on in 'glamour' and 'soft-porn' magazines has reacted on the self-image of Western man and, of course, woman. It has led to dissatisfaction with the living body that falls so far short of its image in paint and on film. To try to compensate for this deficiency, women stuff their breasts with silicone, get their noses straightened and so on. Men to a lesser extent emulate them. The phrase 'plastic fantastic', popular a few years ago in America for describing a heavily remodelled person, accurately suggests that what is aimed at is not humanity but the 'live nude'. It is an unwholesome trend but as medicine and surgery get ever more subtle and potent there is little doubt that it will increase. Just as clothes, used as decoration, can be either lavishly and garishly abundant or disarmingly, deceptively simple, so the plastic recreation of the body itself expresses extremes. While some women pump their breasts full of silicone – thereby risking cancer – others starve themselves, risking annorexic death. While some men build their muscles to uncomfortable proportions, others feel that they will be most attractive if they are lean and hungry. But constant concern with thinness seems to be more a woman's obsession. The diet-conscious woman has a 'figure', not a body. As the pounds of flesh disappear, so too does the vitality, the reality of the flesh. Many see themselves in somewhat the same light as they see the meat they buy from the butchers – in terms of pounds and ounces. But, in the case of Western urban woman, the less she weighs, the more expensive she is likely to be.

It is essentially, (albeit in less extreme form) the tradition of the 'live nude' which so incenses Germaine Greer: 'What happened to woman in painting happened to her in poetry as well. Her beauty was celebrated in terms of the riches which clustered around her: her hair was gold wires, her brow ivory ... She was for consumption.' Later she explodes: 'She absolutely must be young, her body hairless, her flesh buoyant, and *she must not have a sexual organ*' [her italics].

Men, too, have been victimized by the Western nude, and all that it implies. They have been driven towards an ideal of knightly beauty and decorum, and suppressed sexuality, which has been just as oppressive for them as it is has been for 'the fair sex'.

> The hair was snow-white and parted in a straight line from brow to crown revealing the scalp below, colourless and smooth as though the skin had rolled away and the enduring skull already lay exposed. The gold rim of the monocle framed a delicately tinted eyelid ... the face was entirely horrible; as ageless as a tortoise and as inhuman; a painted and smirking obscene travesty ...

The description is of a corpse after cosmetic embalming and is taken from Evelyn Waugh's black comedy *The Loved One*, which is largely concerned with a Los Angeles 'garden of rest'. It might be said that the prettified corpse represents the ultimate expression of the 'prosperous' Western nude. Starting with one element in the multifarious Greek aesthetic celebration of life, the nude pursues its career through the marvellous, idealized forms of Renaissance painting and sculpture, sinks to the debased status, in our culture, of the 'pin-up' and the plastic fantastic and is ultimately consigned to the earth or the flames still decked in the idealized applications which mask the fact that every human body is, invariably after its prime, and often throughout its experience on earth, 'huddled and defenceless'. According to Seymour Fisher:

> ... it may not be a coincidence that the two things we keep most secret from our children are birth and death. Somehow, we do not want them to be directly confronted with how they were created or how they will be extinguished. Perhaps the beginning and the end are linked in their common reference to the fact that there are boundaries to the state of being alive. There is a time of body existence and a time of body non-existence. To master the fear generated by this bare statement has strained the ingenuity of every known society.

The nude can be seen as an attempted solution to the problem. It substitutes for the perishable, disease-prone, unruly body that is pierced with apertures having what may be considered unpleasant purposes a timeless image of ideal proportion. This 'glamour', originally meaning enchantment, is stretched like a skin over Western culture. It encompasses our social life, architecture, all cultural forms – even our weaponry, which is increasingly described as 'sophisticated'. It has been at the expense of the 'naked'. It has meant banishing the real symbols of naked man, the genitals, from overt view. It is no accident that when senior policemen talk about eliminating the 'real filth', they mean representations of copulation, the act of creation. Copulation implies life and change and disease and discomfort and death. It must not be allowed to infect the great nude which is Western society.

But there are hopeful signs that we are moving out of this era. In art, true nakedness is making a reappearance. In thought and culture, a new sense of the natural world is developing. In this century, artists and anthropologists have made enormous contributions towards reacquainting us with our human roots, and electronic media spread the broader understanding far and wide.

THE BATH

The body cannot be suppressed. There have been periods of history, chiefly in the Christian West, when strenuous attempts have been made to remove its appearance and functions from general awareness but those very aspects of the body which have provoked theological and moral censure have ensured that it can never be durably banished.

The bath is perhaps the place where the body, in concealed societies, surfaces most conspicuously. In the urban West at least, two assumptions about the bath and its function are held, both of which are, historically speaking, fallacies. A modern American or European thinks of the bath as basically private and intended for cleansing the body. As a corollary, a cleansed body is regarded as intrinsically desirable, and even essential for health. In fact, most bathing through the ages has been communal and, while cleanliness, or more often perhaps an ideal of cleanliness, has been one aspiration, quite as important have been social and religious factors, as well as notions of well-being unconnected with the removal of dirt.

Modern tub-bathing (although it means ultimately wallowing in a pool containing one's own dirt) is probably more beneficial than harmful, but the equation between cleanliness and health and dirt and disease is not nearly as direct as most people think.

In many parts of the world, water was regarded as a magically purifying agent before it came to be seen as a physically purifying one. It is hard for modern urban man, who secures endless fresh water by turning a tap, to appreciate how precious the substance is. Most inhabitants of the earth have found difficulty, often extreme, in securing a reliable source of water and even then it has often meant daily hard labour for man and beast to convey it to their homes. The 'divine' or 'magical' potency of water was as obvious as that of the sun. Water was vital to every living thing, including man. It made crops grow. The attempted securing of rainfall by propitiation of the gods is one of the oldest supernatural rites. Christian baptism is not a Christian invention but an appropriation of much earlier rituals for sealing man's salvation by contact with the holiness of water. Even today, some of the magical attributes of water linger on. There is, in Christian societies, a feeling that it is virtuous to bathe and that 'cleanliness is next to godliness'.

In hot and dry areas water naturally achieved a special sanctity. The Greeks deified springs. Heaven, as described in the Koran, is essentially a water-garden, replete with willing female bath attendants, who, in fact, are prominent throughout the history of bathing. Like James Bond, ancient Egyptian Pharaohs enjoyed the pleasant relaxation of being massaged by girls after a bath.

Public baths were used by the ancient Greeks and Egyptians but it was left to the Romans, as a direct consequence of that genius for civil engineering which provided imperial Rome with an abundance of water superior to that enjoyed by modern London, to elevate their construction to the proportion of temples. Indeed, the larger Roman bath-houses dwarfed most temples. It became a prestige requirement of emperors to supply ever grander public baths, just as in more devout ages rulers raised churches and cathedrals.

The baths of Caracalla, Rome, completed in the year AD 217, covered an area of some 1100 square feet, which is more than six times the area of St Paul's Cathedral in London. They could accommodate 1600 bathers at a time. According to Gibbon, 'The walls of the lofty apartments were covered in curious mosaic . . . The Egyptian granite was beautifully incrusted with the precious green marble of Numidia.' Baths, to a modern reader, suggest a row of cubicles containing tubs. The Roman baths were nothing like this. They were, in the first place, communal. Moreover, bathing was not simple immersion and drying but an elaborate series of thermal and aqueous experiences which might last all day. Establishments like the Baths of Caracalla were equipped with hot rooms, cold rooms, tepid rooms, with plunge, swimming and individual baths at varying temperatures, with games rooms, massage rooms and annointing rooms. They might also include libraries and restaurants. They were, in fact, civic amenity centres to which admission could be obtained, according to Gibbon, by 'the meanest Roman . . . with a small copper coin'. The later baths of Diocletian held twice as many bathers. They were of such incredible proportions that, a thousand years after they had fallen into ruin, Michelangelo converted the vestibule alone into the great Church of Santa Maria degli Angeli. When Constantine established Christianity as the official religion of the Empire in the early fourth century, he closed the bath-houses. There were then no fewer than a thousand of them in the city of Rome.

Constantine closed the baths because they had become, quite literally, sinks of depravity. According to G.R. Scott: 'The hot baths, in particular, were patronized daily by the most profligate sections of Roman society.' And not only in Rome itself: in the provincial baths, according to Seneca, people drank and gambled and 'in addition to every ordinary form of vulgarity and obscenity, they practised immoralities that can only be hinted at'. And yet the institution of public baths in Rome was originally the product of hygienic and ethical considerations of the loftiest kind.

The original regulations governing conduct in bath-houses were very strict. Men and women were segregated. Parents were not permitted to bathe with their own children or a father-in-law with his own son-in-law. Various experiments were attempted to maintain high standards of conduct. These included bizarre ones like the appointment of eunuchs as attendants at the women's baths and Draconian ones like making it a capital offence for a male to force an entry into the women's baths. But, relentlessly, the inevitable erotic overtones of the situation imposed themselves, until mixed nude bathing became customary. The subsequent history of the Roman baths, up to the time of Constantine, is that of so many human institutions: reform, followed by renewed slide into corruption. G.R. Scott says:

> The morality of the baths was dependent upon the whim of the reigning monarch. Some emperors, dissolute themselves, had no scruples of any kind. Thus Gallienus not only allowed the sexes to bathe together in all their nudity but was himself a regular frequenter of the thermae, where, stripped to the buff, he joined in the game with gusto, bathing with the women . . .

Domitian countenanced mixed bathing, Marcus Aurelius prohibited it. So did Hadrian. So did Trajan. So did Alexander Severus. Heliogabalus restored it in all its old-time vigour. So the pendulum swung until, in the end, the first Christian Emperor of Rome abolished the institution forever.

The essence of the problem facing the Roman authorities, and indeed inherent in the human personality of those authorities, is neatly caught by these two passages of Scott:

> It is significant that the most luxurious and magnificent days of the termae, and the years when they were at the height of their popularity, were coincident with those periods when promiscuity and nudity in bathing were either expressly permitted or tolerated.

> At no period were nudity and promiscuity obligatory. Even when mixed bathing was at its height, there were apartments where those blessed with some remnants of modesty could [go in order to be] free from the embarrassing presence of members of the other sex or the nude members of their own sex.

Most people, if given the choice, do not seem to want freedom from 'the embarrassing presence of members of the other sex'. Indeed, they will flock to places where it is available, and if such places also afford the opportunity for naked intercourse (in every sense) with members of the opposite sex their popularity is assured. The lure of the body will always triumph over the prevailing morality – given half a chance anyway. And the body's legitimate requirements will always ensure that the body itself re-emerges from banishment. Public baths are, even in the eyes of a strict moralist, a desirable facility. A brothel is categorically undesirable. The trouble is that the former has an almost ineluctable tendency to evolve into the latter.

The history of European bath-houses in many ways duplicates that of the Roman, with the grandeur and, often, the truly hygienic factors, removed and the sensual ones, if anything, augmented.

It is perhaps worth pointing out, at this stage, that the baths of both Rome and Europe fulfilled a genuine social need. They provided places of congregation and relaxation. True, in their decadent phases they purveyed erotic diversion but they also played the part of community centres where people could meet, eat, play and talk as well as flirt and bathe.

Europe lived for six hundred years with the ruins of Roman civil engineering and domestic architecture. Aqueducts crumbled slowly (although stretches of them remain to this day as testimony to the excellence of the Roman engineers). Baths fell into disuse. Villas, circuses and bath-houses were plundered for stone. The tradition of baths and bathing was lost. Its loss was facilitated by the hostility of the early Church to water. St Jerome actually congratulated nuns on being lousy and for never allowing water to touch their persons. It was, in fact, only the late Protestant work ethic, with its acceptance of the human body as raw material for labour in the service of the Lord, which re-hallowed cleanliness.

Charlemagne is credited with the initial rediscovery, in the eighth century, of the virtues of bathing. He is reported to have heard that much benefit attended immersion in the springs of Aix-la-Chapelle. He visited them and was converted. He went on to build a great bathhouse in the grounds of his own palace, which duly became the scene of debauchery.

To Charlemagne, therefore, may be credited not only the revival of the tradition of public baths but also the foundation of the spa in Europe. The word derives from the name of a Belgian town where there were natural springs. It came to mean a resort containing a natural source of water credited with beneficial powers. Originally, these powers were considered to be miraculous rather than medicinal, but as medicine inched towards being a science (a condition it perhaps only fully achieved in the present century) spa waters were credited with therapeutic powers. It was, for obvious reasons, desirable for such waters to have properties which distinguished them from ordinary, run-of-the-stream water. The chief qualities suitable for this purpose were variations of temperature and of taste. Thus natural hot springs and springs of water that had a 'mineral' taste were hailed as being sovereign remedies for virtually every ailment known. The Romans, of course, had used natural sources of water, in England. But the Romans had sensibly regarded natural springs as a handy aid in the construction of their customary bathing facilities, rather than as magical sources of virtue.

But, once again, as in Roman times, spas formed centres of resort and social activity and, as an almost inevitable corollary, of erotic diversion. All spas seem to have undergone the Roman oscillation between relative permissiveness and relative strictness although few seem to have become mere aquatic orgies. The town of Bath itself permitted mixed bathing for centuries though not nude mixed bathing. Still, fun and games were obviously quite as much an attraction as shaking off 'cold humours', as the following eighteenth-century account suggests:

> Handsome japanned bowls floated before the ladies, laden with confectionery, or with oils, essences, and perfumery for their use.

Now and then one of these bowls would float away from its owner, and her swain would float after it, bring it again before her, and, if he were in the humour, would turn on his back and affect to sink to the bottom, out of mere rapture at the opportunity of serving her.

Spas were essentially the preserve of the upper classes who could afford to travel to them. There have always been classes of itinerant poor but, until quite recently, travel was largely the privilege of the well-to-do. The great bulk of the populace, therefore, could never frolic in a natural spring but they did, from about the twelfth century onwards, start to demand bathing facilities. These were catered for by the institution, common throughout Europe, of 'sweating' baths, originally from Russia and North Europe, whose familiar name is still one for a place of low resort, the 'stews'. There was no Roman grandeur about the stews and not much real health either. They were normally filthy and vermin-ridden. They usually consisted of wooden buildings containing huge stoves which were used to heat large stones. Water was regularly thrown over the stones and the bathers basked in the resulting steam. Again, conditions varied, but mixed, nude bathing was common and some of the stews were equipped with eating and sleeping facilities. According to Scott, these 'sweating baths were little more than brothels. They were the meeting places for the most depraved, immoral and libidinous characters to be found in all London town.' In the reign of Henry VIII, because of the rampant spread of venereal diseases, they were closed.

In the eighteenth century they started up again, supplemented by the new Turkish baths of which Casanova, visiting London at this period, said: 'A rich man can sup, bathe and sleep with a fashionable courtesan ... it makes a magnificent debauch and only costs six guineas.'

The truth is that, in a concealed culture where sex is either barely tolerated within defined relationships or actively deprecated, and the naked human body is rarely seen, the public bath will inevitably succumb to dammed-up eroticism. This will lead to reform and banning. But then the practical value of the baths will result in their reappearance. This cycle is inescapable. In England, at the present day, the proliferation of so-called saunas (actually closer to tiny, electric Turkish baths than the steamy Finnish and Russian archetype) and their increasing decline into brothels demonstrates that the mechanism is still in good working order. We may anticipate, since there is no sign of any fundamental change in attitudes to the body and sexuality, that the saunas will be closed down before very long, especially since the next swing towards an erotic outlet has already made an appearance – naked sea-bathing.

Naturally, the oscillation between permissiveness and repression has no metronomic regularity. The intervals between peaks vary and, indeed, different phases of the cycle overlap both temporally and geographically. Surprising juxtapositions are found. Thus, in mid-Victorian England, when the body was perhaps least tolerated, not only did prostitution flourish but there were curious anomalies in people's attitudes to nakedness. The bathing-suit had not yet been invented and sea-bathing was becoming fashionable. The Reverend Francis Kilvert, noted in his diary that at Weston-Super-Mare in 1872: 'There was a delicious feeling of freedom in stripping in the open air and running down naked to the sea, where ... the red morning sunshine (was) glowing upon the naked limbs of the bathers.' At Sandown, two years later, he beheld: 'One beautiful girl ... entirely naked on the sand ... She seemed a Venus Anadyomene fresh risen from the waves.' But at nearby Shanklin he noted with disgust that 'one has to adopt the detestable custom of bathing in drawers'.

Perhaps surprisingly, the true delights of bathing seem to be most fully appreciated by people who live in unconcealed and relatively unsupressed cultures. The Polynesians rejoiced in bathing. It was normal for them to bathe two or three times a day. The Japanese, who traditionally felt no shame about the body and little about sex, have a long tradition of bathing which has not been widely reported to have degenerated into debauchery. Rather it has acquired a mystique of almost spiritual virtue. The following is from an account given recently by a Japanese man:

> Bathing of the Japanese may be certainly called washing of the life rather than cleaning of the body ... At the moment when they begin to sing a popular song cheerfully in the bathroom, any of them is no more a carpenter, a cart coolie, nor a navvy, but now he is a poet ... Bathing washes away their discontent, and their disposition as labourers is melted away in the bath-box; they are converted to optimists ...

In Japan, the sexes were often segregated, but not rigidly. A curtain or low wall might divide the men's from the women's section. In spite of the relative 'naturalness' of the baths in Japan, it is interesting that Banto or bath boys were kept busy scrubbing down the women, just as in the baths of ancient Greece. There is no doubt that each sex derives keen satisfaction from being attended in the bath by the other.

If the bath has, historically, been a place of physical, spiritual or erotic utility and pleasure, rather than a necessity, there is another sanitary facility which our basic physiological process renders inescapable. I quote from the initial lines of Alexander Kira's admirable treatise, *The Bathroom,* which, while essentially a manual for those professionally concerned with the subject (architects, designers etc.) is rich in both information and wisdom.

> Man has always and everywhere been faced with the same fundamental problems of personal hygiene that concern us today. The ways in which he has coped with them have, however, varied enormously . . . by far the most important determinants have been our various philosophical, psychological and religious attitudes regarding . . . the body, sex, birth, death, illness, menstruation, elimination and cleansing. Virtually the only absolutes in this entire area of human existence have been those natural and involuntary bodily processes over which we have no control whether we like the facts or not.

Elimination of wastes is a great, and largely unsung, fact of human, and indeed all animal, life. Basically it involves what are politely known as defecation and urination. Menstruation is, of course, a third manifestation but it is intermittent, confined to one sex and has been discussed earlier in this book. 'Going to the lavatory' is a daily, almost hourly, event and yet it remains almost a taboo subject. It is, however, of great interest, psychologically, historically and practically. Discussing it is hampered by, among other things, the fact that there is no easy vocabulary. In man's mental flight from his own physiology, he endlessly fabricates euphemisms to distance himself from unwelcome facts. As each euphemism becomes too familiar, and hence apparently blunt, a new one is piled on top. Although 'lavatory' means etymologically a place for washing, it will be used here to mean a place for elimination. There is simply *no* generally accepted and unambiguous alternative. 'Privy' is perhaps the best but it is, by now, quaint.

The first lavatory was that shared with all the beasts of the field, the wide earth itself. Simple man can indeed still manifest a totally unselfconscious attitude towards elimination, though most primitives at least go off alone away from habitations to defecate. A Tartar curse was: 'I would thou mightest tarry so long in one place that thou mightest smell thine own dung as the Christians do!'

Reasonably well-off citizens of modern cities, whether Christian or not, have largely been relieved of the necessity of smelling their own dung. A contemporary domestic lavatory, especially if fitted with fan-extractors, ensures that little olfactory evidence of the daily necessity to empty the body of food residues remains. Of course, even privileged citizens are not always at home and it is likely that everyone still experiences unsatisfactory public facilities from time to time which bring an inescapable reminder of the perpetual physiological process and its disagreeable final product. The achievement of modern urban sanitation has been one of the most titanic tasks human technology has ever undertaken. There is little doubt that the great majority of those who profess disgust with the modern world and keen nostalgia for more gracious, elegant or noble ages would receive a severe shock if they could be translated back to their favoured period. Does he or she yearn for the stylish world of Restoration comedy? Oxford antiquary, Anthony à Wood, after Charles II and his court had spent the summer of 1665 in his city, noted in his diary: 'Though they were neat and gay in their apparel, yet they were very nasty and beastly, leaving at their departure their excrements in every corner, in chimneys, studies, coalhouses, cellars.' Does the splendour of Louis XIV's court arouse restrospective yearning? A court lady wrote:

> At Fontainebleau, one must wait for darkness to use the open spaces. This grieved Her Grace, who preferred privacy and something to sit on. She found the streets of Fontainebleau full of reminders of a human frailty she deplored, and especially of souvenirs of the Swiss Guards.

Throughout most of the 'civilized', or urban ages, the great majority of people have had to live on uncomfortably intimate terms with their own dung. Of course, while the prevailing sanitary conditions, or lack of them, would strike a modern very forcibly, as they do when he visits part of the world where conditions are still primitive, the people of the time accepted them as normal. Complaints such as the above are rare. Literature, with a very few exceptions, hardly ever mentions excretion. How such a repellently conspicuous part of life could have left so few cultural traces is suggested by V.S. Naipaul, writing about modern India:

> Indians defecate everywhere. They defecate, mostly beside the railway tracks. But they also defecate on the beaches; they defecate on the streets; they never look for cover ... These squatting figures ... are never spoken of; they are never written about; they

are not mentioned in novels or stories . . . the truth is that Indians do not see these squatters and might even, with complete sincerity, deny that they exist.

The story of man's struggle with his own dung is wittily and exhaustively recounted in Lawrence Wright's *Clean and Decent*. Almost all of it is depressing and sordid, the history of inadequate measures, taken too late, and of indescribable conditions and epidemics. Although the Romans had underground sewers, many later towns until the last century had exposed sewers running down the streets and the only recourse with domestic soil was to empty it out of a window. Wright includes strange and picturesque manifestations such as the Edinburgh functionary whose stock in trade was a bucket and great cloak for the comfort of pedestrians 'caught short' a long way from home, for there were, of course, no public conveniences. He describes the 'easing stools' made to resemble a pile of books but, so that aspirant users should not mistake them for real books, always with the same titles, either *Mystères de Paris* or *Voyage au Pays Bas*. Wright reports that kings and generals have received embassies while seated on 'pierced thrones' and the ambassadors have been proud of the honour. More dismally, he makes it clear that romantic moated castles were really reeking prisons surrounded by rings of sewage, and reveals that, after thousands of years of this struggle, conditions in some parts of London in Victoria's age probably represented a nadir. The inhabitants of certain pockets on small tributaries of the Thames lived in wooden houses built over what were in effect open sewers, which were their sole source of *drinking water*!

The modern way with excrement is to treat the anus as merely marking one stage in dung's progress towards the open sea. The network of pipes and sewers under a modern city represents a kind of artificial extension of the intestinal tract conveying a city's dung away from the city. It is far from satisfactory because the dung remains a pollutant which must somewhere have its effect. The sensible solution would be to process it and use it as fertilizer. But it is virtually impossible for modern Western human beings to be sensible about their own excrement. This was strikingly demonstrated in the preparations for the American Apollo programme for putting a man on the moon. Not only did the media ignore the rather obvious problem confronting men in space suits but NASA itself was reluctant to broach it. According to Kira, 'It wasn't until 1968, after bitter crew complaints . . . that a major conference involving NASA and contractor personnel was held on the subject.' The Apollo programme revealed just how profound is man's psychological revulsion from his chief bodily product. It was decreed that while liquid waste (urine) could be ejected from the travelling space craft, solid wastes must not be. The feeling was that public opinion would not stand for the polluting of the solar system with a few human turds, even though they would, in fact, have been instantly dispersed in the form of atomic particles.

Defecation, to the conscious mind of civilized man, is an unpleasant necessity and its product categorically offensive. But, as psychology has long since made clear, to the infant mind, it is exciting and pleasurable, and feces are a wondrous creation. The final attitude of the adult is thus inescapably ambivalent and there are some who react to the taboo against enjoyment and interest in the act of defecation, as some do against any taboo, by finding the forbidden fruit irresistible. According to Havelock Ellis:

> In Parisian brothels provision is made for those who are sexually excited by the spectacle of the act of defecation by means of a 'tabouret de verre', from under the glass floor of which, the spectacle of the defecating woman may be closely observed.

We have concealed the body beneath clothing and provided secret places, supported by monumental technology, for the exercise of its eliminatory functions but it is essentially a cosmetic exercise. While urban sanitation is clearly a good thing, the denial of the body and its processes is psychologically harmful. We can only build a harmonious culture on the basis of reality, and excrement is an important part of our reality.

'Love has pitched his mansion in the place of excrement', the poet W.B. Yeats noted sourly. Other writers have been considerably more indignant at what might seem to have been the mind of the practical joker at work on the construction of the human body. Jonathan Swift found the inextricable union of sexual allure and excretion utterly intolerable. 'But Celia, Celia, Celia,' he lamented, 'shits'. It is, in fact, almost impossible not to experience some degree of confusion, which may reach schizophrenic proportions, at the consideration that love and excrement are so nearly commingled.

'Walter,' the pseudonymous Victorian author of the massive erotic journal *My Secret Life* encountered a woman who, although a prostitute, was extremely reluctant to copulate. Questioned, she complained that it was a poor thing to be a woman and have to allow men 'to put their muck into us'. 'Walter' reflected ruefully that this was not a very nice way to consider the seed of life. But it is, in fact, a psychologically inescapable way. Sperm, urine, feces, babies and menstrual discharges inevitably become confused in the undisciplined depths of the mind and lend each other special resonances and metaphorical values. The origin of the sense that pervades our culture that man is a centaur, half god and half brute, mind among the stars and feet deep in the clay, is largely conditioned by the fact that excretion and physical love have the same bodily focus.

LADY GODIVA

It was originally with reluctance that the name of the Countess Godiva of Mercia was appropriated to head this chapter. The requirement was for a lady, famous in history or legend, who could represent all the women who have exposed their bodies in clothed cultures. Clearly this class would be largely composed of ladies of, at best, dubious virtue, grading from prostitutes to actresses. Should a pious Saxon wife, celebrated historically for the foundation of monasteries, be put in the vanguard of this army? Other names were canvassed: Aphrodite, Goddess of Desire, born of the foam seething from the severed genitals of Uranus; the Empress Theodora of Byzantium who emerged from the red light district to rule (with her husband Justinian) the Empire, but retained her delight in giving lewd stage performances; Thais, the whore of Athens, or even – although the plunge to modern commercial coquetry is inevitably bathetic – Gypsy Rose Lee, the archetypal strip-tease artiste? None of them, nor any other that came to mind, evoked the essential image of a naked woman among clothed men. It is ironic that the name of the virtuous British aristocrat has become inextricably linked with the idea of body display, while her laudable deeds are little remembered. Lady Godiva has become a universal symbol of the naked body.

The historical Lady Godiva was the devout wife of Earl Leofric of Mercia and was instrumental in founding a number of religious houses including, in 1043, a Benedictine monastery at Coventry. But the exploit which made her name immortal is legendary although, like many legends, it may have a basis in fact. The story goes that the good countess, distressed by the burden of taxation levied by her greedy husband, implored him to ease the burden on the poor. When the Earl could no longer ignore her importunity, he agreed, on condition that she ride naked through Coventry. This was, of course, intended to be an impossible condition which would dispose of the matter permanently. He had failed to reckon with his wife's mettle. She gave instructions that everyone in the village should remain indoors with shutters secured, then removed all her clothes, mounted her horse and rode down the main street. The villagers respected her instructions – with the exception of a particular tailor, for whom the lure proved too great. Peeping Tom parted his shutters and enjoyed the spectacle, whereupon a just providence struck him blind. Leofric, confounded, fulfilled his part of the bargain and the oppressive taxes were lifted.

In fact, nakedness in eleventh-century England, where the great hall of the castle was likely to be the only warm room, was far from uncommon and the contemporary force of the story derives largely from the rank of the lady. It was the fact that an aristocrat rendered herself vulnerable before the common people that supplied the coercive power of the deed. Nonetheless, for our purposes, the tale contains most of the essential ingredients of the long history of sexual repression and its often pitiable consequences. We are told, for example, that Lady Godiva was not *totally* naked. She possessed exquisite long hair which hung about her but, doubtless stirred by the breeze and the movements of her mount, permitted her limbs to be tantilizingly glimpsed. Then again, she did not walk, which would have immediately rendered her ordinary and slightly pathetic. No, she rode. She was on display, raised as if on a stage, an object for inspection. Walking, her movements would have been functionally dictated. Riding, she would have been forced to carry herself in a particular way, her comportment presumably dictated by modesty, insofar as the situation permitted, but nevertheless calculated like a performer's. The horse itself would have been an actor in the erotic show, privileged to feel its mistress's naked limbs on its flanks. Animals, employed with delicacy or elemental crudity, have often figured in erotic entertainments. The tasteful artiste decks herself in a flock of doves. The Marseilles whore copulates with a donkey. But Lady Godiva's ride would have been deprived of its key resonances, which have kept it fresh to this day, without the indispensable participation of the unfortunate Peeping Tom. In his utter inability to resist the chance of seeing an attractive naked woman, he stands for all the men who, throughout the ages, have flocked to brothels and burlesque shows, both of which, in some form or another, are ineradicable in concealed societies. The tailor was not, apparently, a monster. He was an ordinary man with an ordinary man's frustrated desires. Since he was visited with terrible retribution, it is reasonable to suppose that he knew in advance that his deed was wrong and that he would have felt miserable and self-reproachful about it. In this too, he stands for the great majority of civilized men who, aware that their sexual misconduct is at best deprecated, at worst utterly proscribed with penalties that have at times been capital, have nonetheless remorsefully obeyed their ineluctable instinctual imperatives. Peeping Tom's blindness symbolizes that blindness to the ideals of civilized society which is inescapable when men give way to their 'baser instincts'. The story of Lady Godiva and Peeping Tom portrays a civilization that has still failed to harmonize its social and spiritual aspirations with the primal instinct.

Lady Godiva's piety which, at first consideration, would seem to distance her from what will essentially be the story of commercial sex, can be seen, from a deeper perspective, to be a natural ingredient. For, as Witkowski and Nass in their exhaustive work *Le Nu au théâtre* point out: 'The origins of the theatre, of prostitution and of the ancient religions are related.' The focal point, from which all three, and many ancillary aspects of human culture, radiate is the sexual act itself. Religion begins with magic and the most magical thing in the universe to primitive minds, after the blatant fact of the tangible universe itself, is the process of generation. The sexual act thus becomes a metaphor for all that is mysterious, and is a powerful coercive act when employed as sympathetic magic. People compel crops to grow by performing acts of virility and fecundity, that is, by copulating in their neighbourhood. All primitive religious ceremonies are rooted in the dance and the dance is invariably erotic and often orgiastic. All movement, growth, power in the cosmos, is assimilated into sexuality. As religion becomes more hieratic and complex, and its tenets acquire an overlay of morality, the primal erotic source becomes obscured. The Virgin Mary, 'spotless Virgin free from stain', is the primal fertility goddess turned upside down. Her purity is as intensely erotic as is Aphrodite's dedication to promiscuity.

It is no wonder that prostitution, now so secular and often sordid, was in its origins religious and exalted. Havelock Ellis gives a 'typical example' of early religious prostitution as originally recorded by Herodotus:

> In the fifth century before Christ, at the temple of Mylitta, the Babylonian Venus ... every woman once in her life had to come and give herself to the first stranger who threw a coin in her lap, in worship of the goddess ... Very similar customs existed in other parts of Western Asia, in North Africa, in Cyprus and other islands of the Eastern Mediterranean, and also in Greece, where the Temple of Aphrodite on the fort at Corinth possessed over a thousand hierodules, dedicated to the service of the goddess, from time to time, as Strabo states, by those who desired to make thank-offering for mercies vouchsafed to them.

True prostitution, in which a woman exchanges sexual favours for pecuniary rewards, is virtually unknown amongst primitives. In its earliest institutionalized forms it is usually associated with religion and the practitioners acquire some of the mystique of priestesses. The mystery of the body, which is an integral part of the experience of primitives, becomes hived off as soon as concealment and sexual repression start to characterize a culture. Once this stage has been reached, prostitution becomes secularized, though even in the West a faint aura of the divine, even if much degraded, still attaches to the profession. Prostitutes are often given, especially in literature, titles suggestive of religion, such as 'abbess' for the madam of a brothel, and names like Magdalene, and Paphian for the girls themselves, while the common terms harlot, whore and strumpet have biblical resonances. A brothel is probably, after a place of worship, and perhaps at some profound level before it, the place most charged with elemental mystery.

According to Havelock Ellis:

> The woman who sells herself for money purely as a professional matter, without any thought of love or passion, and who, by virtue of her profession, belongs to a pariah class definitely and rigidly excluded from the main body of her sex, is a phenomenon which can seldom be found except in developed civilization. It is altogether incorrect to speak of prostitutes as a mere survival from primitive times.

Prostitution is generated by the repression of sexuality and, in concealed and repressed societies, cannot be abolished. Its history echoes the history of other aspects of sexual expression in cultures which condemn it, an oscillation. But institutions which require bricks and mortar, such as public baths, can, if with difficulty, be extirpated. Prostitution, which in its simplest form has no need of anything but purchaser and seller, is harder to deal with. Obviously there are no exact statistics available which describe the exact ratio of number of prostitutes to degree of repression, but the available literature suggests strongly that in concealed societies prostitution is a constant and, in its quantitative expression, is little affected by repressive measures. Its tactics and techniques may change, but the grand strategy triumphs everywhere. I recall, when I first returned to England from the United States in the final year of the Second World War, being surprised to find the streets bordering Hyde Park lined, at intervals of fifty yards or so, with girls soliciting passing cars. The *Street Offences Act* of 1959 swept them off the streets and put them at the ends of telephone lines. The era of the call girl had, in London anyway, arrived. The penalties for prostitution, and prostitution-related offences, have sometimes been savage. Reccared, a sixth-century Visigoth king, punished prostitutes with three hundred lashes and expulsion from the city. Justinian exiled panders on pain of death. The French king and saint, Louis IX, banished prostitutes from France and seized all their property, even clothing. But when he went on crusade in the East he found prostitutes plying their trade in the very shadow of his tent.

Havelock Ellis writes:

> In 1560 an edict of Charles IX abolished brothels, but the number of prostitutes was thereby increased rather than diminished, while many new kinds of brothels appeared in unsuspected shapes and were more dangerous than the more recognized brothels which had been suppressed.

This expresses a perennial dilemma confronting civil, and sometimes religious authorities: whether to attempt to control prostitution or to eradicate it. Again and again, the fact is borne in on governments that, since prostitution exists it should be incorporated in the civil administration so that it can be supervised and kept reasonably healthy by means of medical inspections. There are state brothels at present in, among other places, West Germany and the American state of Nevada. The inevitable next step is an outcry from moralists that the state is playing the part of bawd. Then legislation is passed to make brothels illegal. The girls are back on the streets, trailing venereal disease. The cycle is remorseless.

Christianity, which more than any other religion has deprecated the flesh and its frailties, might have been expected to wage unceasing war on prostitution. In fact, its attitude to the institution has been approximately that of secular authorities. Undoubtedly, the chief reason is that, at a level not often admitted even by its own theoreticians, Christianity has perceived that the maintenance of its influence through the sacraments, which chiefly concern the regulation of erotic matters, would be threatened without prostitution, the inevitable concomitant of sexual repression. It could almost be said that Christianity, as an institution rather than as a doctrine, is rooted in sexual repression. The priest and the prostitute could be seen almost as its twin pillars. Nevertheless, the Church has made intermittent attempts to eradicate prostitution. The issue has often been further complicated by the fact that the Church has rarely been above deriving an income from the leasing of property to be used for immoral purposes. London is still full of mini-brothels operating in property owned by the Church. The Church as an institution, that group of human beings, predominantly male and often vowed to celibacy, has also had more personal contact with prostitution. For a variety of reasons, the Church has never felt that it could safely make an all-out assault on an institution which might seem to represent the antithesis of all it represented. It has in practice, if not in formal admission, appeared to acknowledge a symbiotic relationship.

Reformers have often argued that the chief basis of prostitution is economic deprivation, and that if women are given the opportunity to earn a reasonable living by other means it will wither away. However, the demand for prostitution is such that women, or at least the more favoured among them, will always be able to earn more as whores. One American girl gave up teaching for prostitution because, she said, society clearly valued her vagina more than her brain, and who was she not to benefit from the disparity in esteem? But perhaps the chief reason why prostitution will never be suppressed by economic reform is that the idealists who propose it ignore the participation of the prostitutes themselves. Slavery can be abolished by legislative action. But then very few slaves enjoy being slaves. Undoubtedly, a lot of prostitutes do enjoy their work. Wilhelm Stekel documents the case of an upper-class girl who ran away to work in a brothel, was found and restored to her family, and vowed to kill herself if she were not allowed to go back to the brothel. Such fanatical devotion to the trade is probably rare, but there is little doubt that the life of leisure, relative wealth and abundant sex appeals to a lot of girls. All commentators, however reluctantly, admit that, as a class, voluntary prostitutes are often as well-balanced and content as housewives or other working girls. 'Walter', while collecting material for his 'secret life', had intercourse with literally thousands of prostitutes, and few of them expressed dismay at their lot. The ones that did tended to be ill-favoured and unsuccessful.

If prostitution is virtually unknown to primitives, proto-theatrical activity is not. Earlier in this book Jane Goodall's description of a 'rain dance' by chimpanzees, witnessed in the wild, was quoted. The most primitive human communities almost invariably include dancing, with percussive accompaniment, as one of the earliest forms of cultural expression. Such dances invariably have a strong erotic component. Brian Hugh Macdermot describes Nuer dances: 'Sometimes lines of dancing women would advance and then retreat, flicking their bottoms upwards in a provocative manner, their leather skirts undulating.' In this primal, orgiastic dance, which is rooted in nature and fertility religion, can be seen the origin of the theatre. Although it is communal, it will necessarily include an audience, the very young, the very old, the exhausted, the sick and perhaps some who prefer the role of spectator to participant. At early paleolithic levels of cultural evolution, the simple dance often evolves into elaborate and stylized rituals which include almost all the elements of fully-developed theatre. The participants may spend days or weeks making gorgeous costumes which often represent stylized figures, gods, goddesses, spirits, animals etc. They create 'sets', that is, specially decorated places within the village compounds. They have 'scripts' or traditional sequences of movement and sometimes of chanting or speech. And they divide the village into audience and performers. One remarkable and well-documented example, which displays on the one hand the attributes of a religious organization and on the other those of a theatrical company and which stems from an early cultural stage, is the 'Arioi' society of Tahiti. The missionaries regarded its members as 'human harpies, in whose characters all that is most loathsome, earthly, sensual, devilish was combined'. But Bengt Daniellson demonstrates that this blinkered view stemmed from a total incomprehension of the roots and purpose of the institution. For one thing, the Arioi's members regarded *themselves* as missionaries, dedicated to the maintenance and spread of their society's most profound religious truths, and every aspirant member had to learn by heart the sacred traditions and songs handed down.

A group of Arioi would arrive in a flotilla of canoes which sometimes contained several thousand men and women. On the host

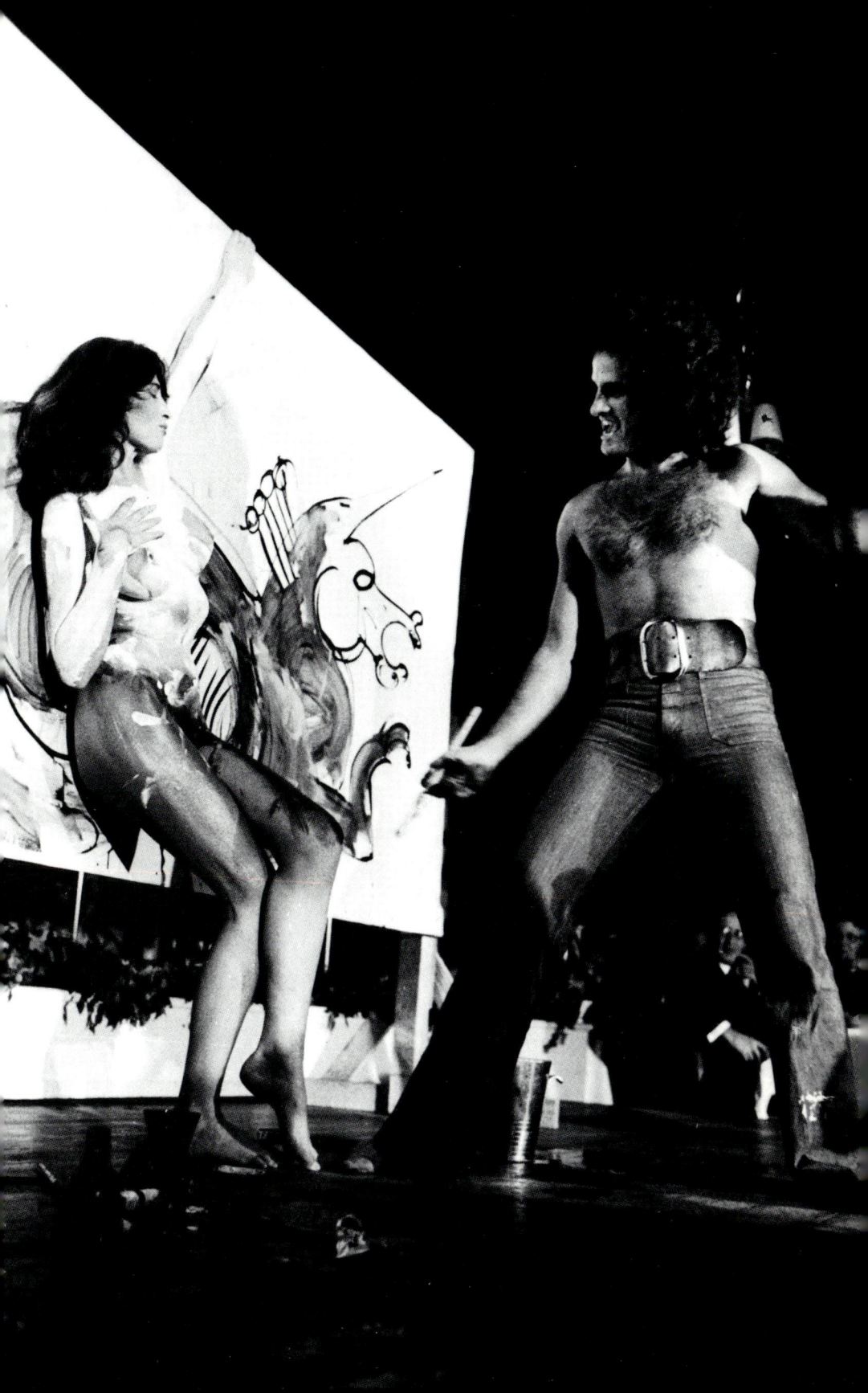

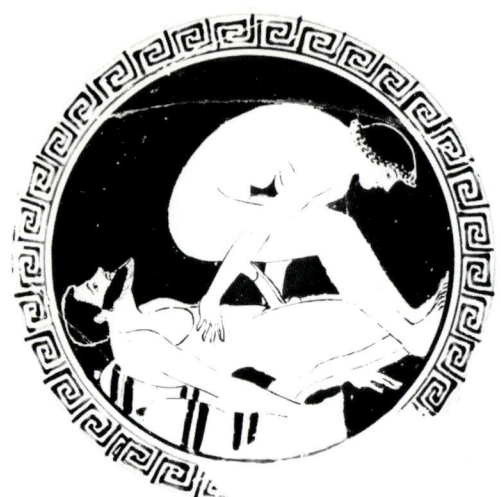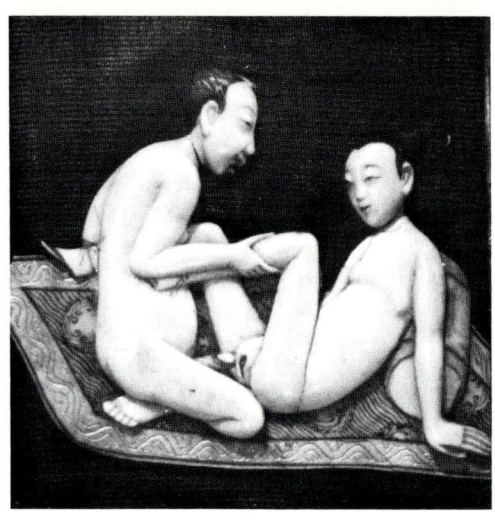

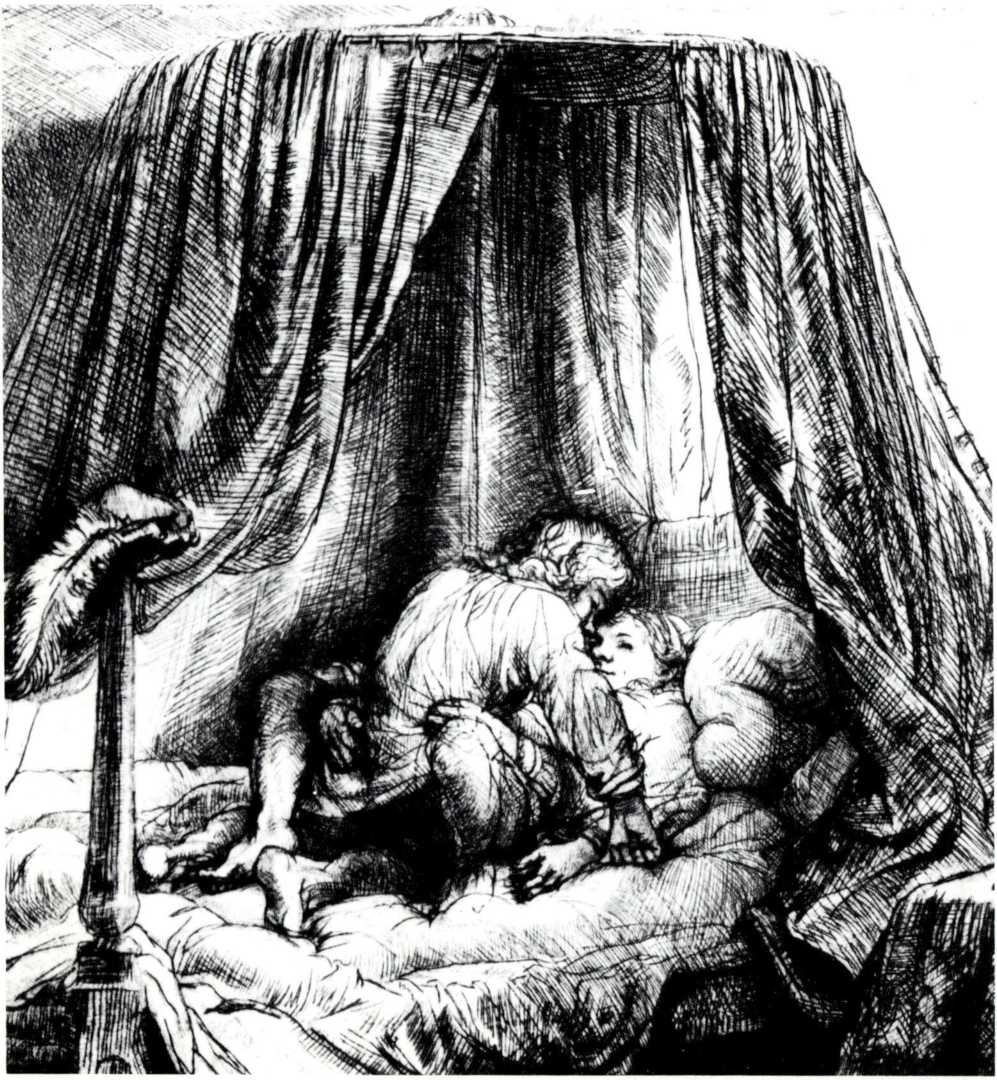

The question of when art becomes eroticism has exercised men's minds for centuries, although it does not seem to be one which has much concerned the artists themselves. The aesthetic qualities of a Greek vase painting or a Chinese ivory carving (left) are held to outweigh their erotic content; and Rembrandt's touching etching (below left) is widely acknowledged to be art. But while the temple carvings at Khajuraho (bottom) are undoubtedly religious art, photographs of them have usually been viewed as pornographic! The paintings of Giulio Romano, the popular sixteenth-century artist (below) appear to have been erotic in their intention. The artist actually applying paint to his subject (previous page) eludes classification along these lines. The only thing which seems certain is that different people see things differently.

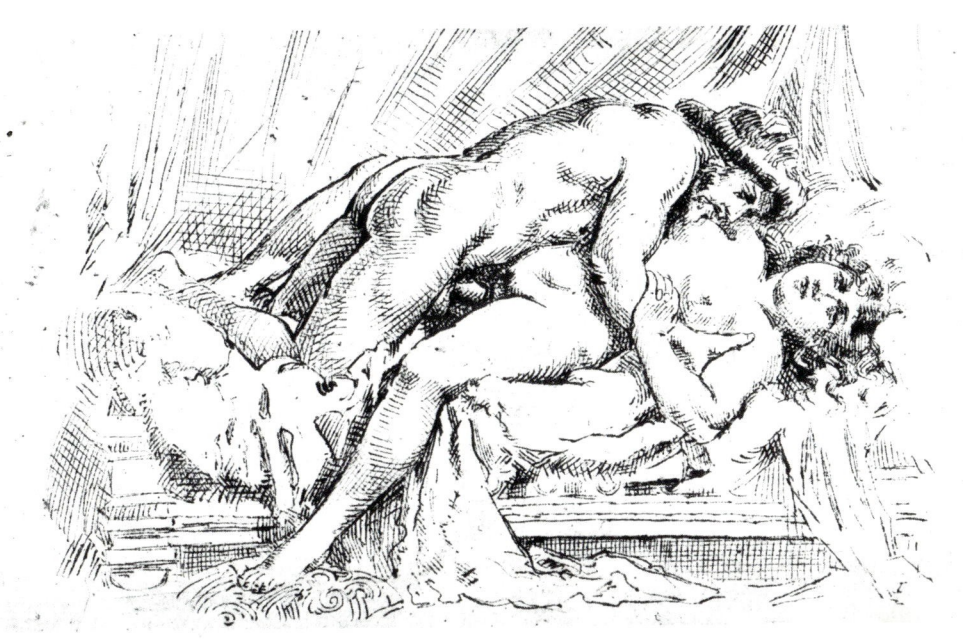

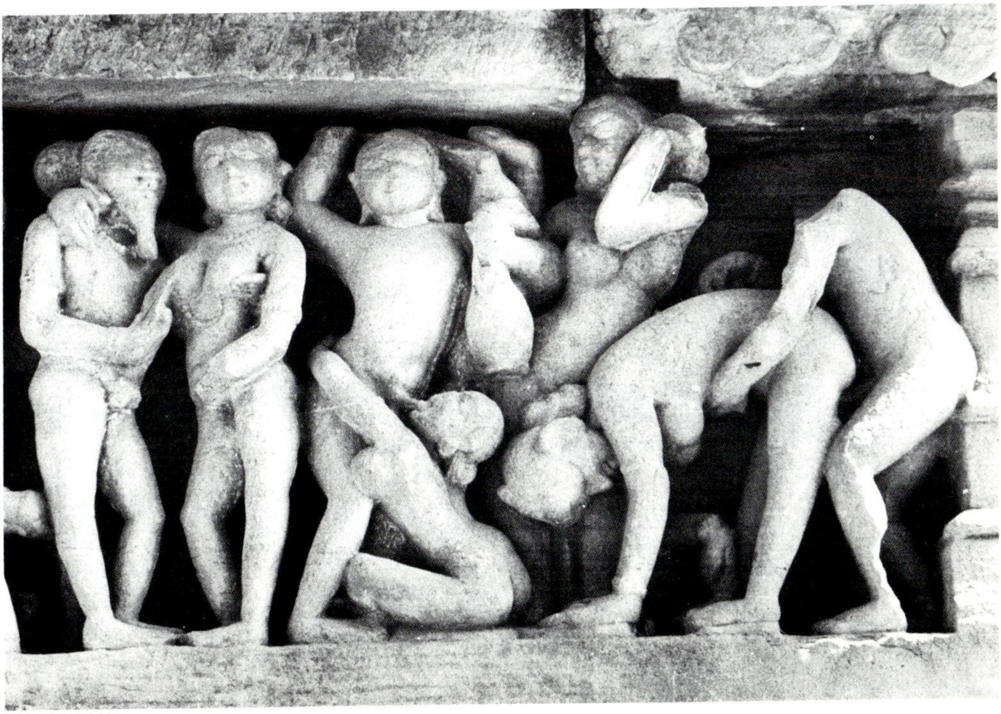

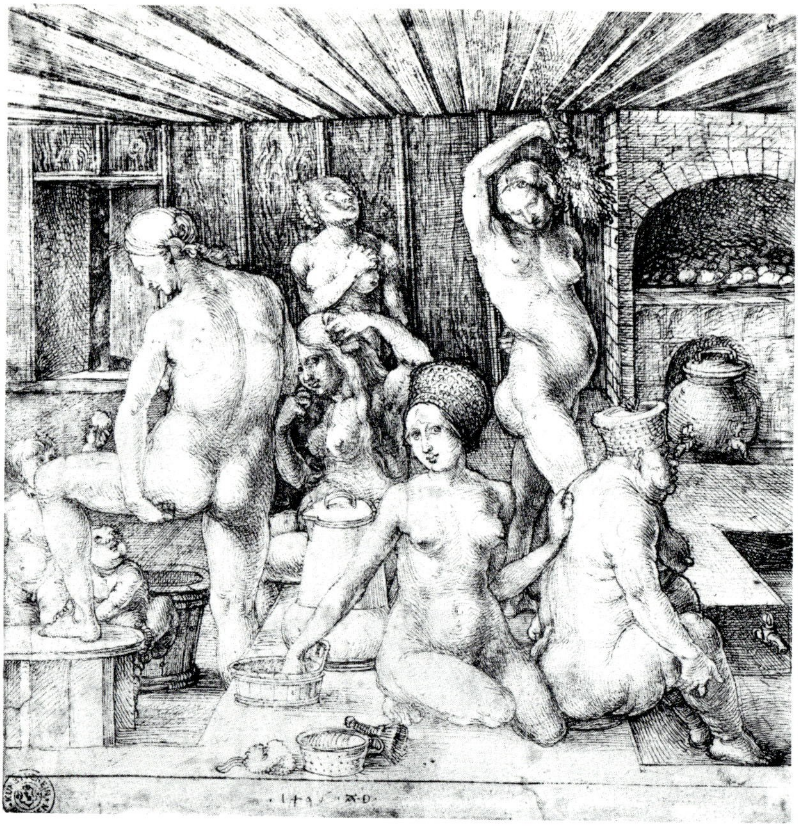

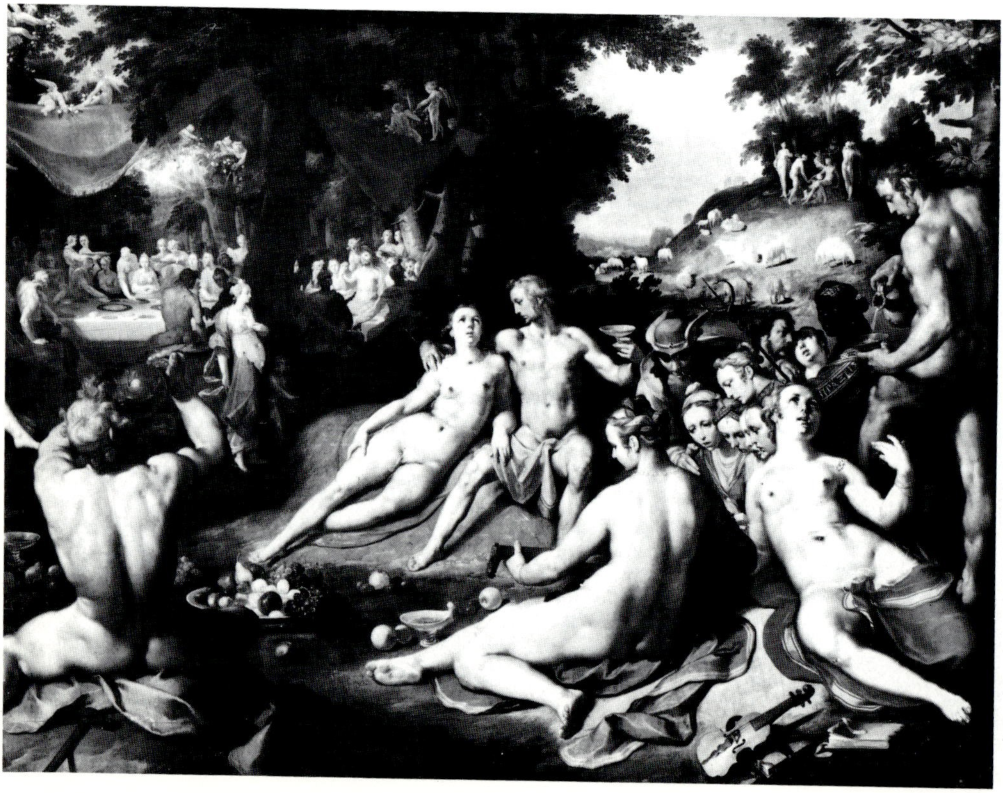

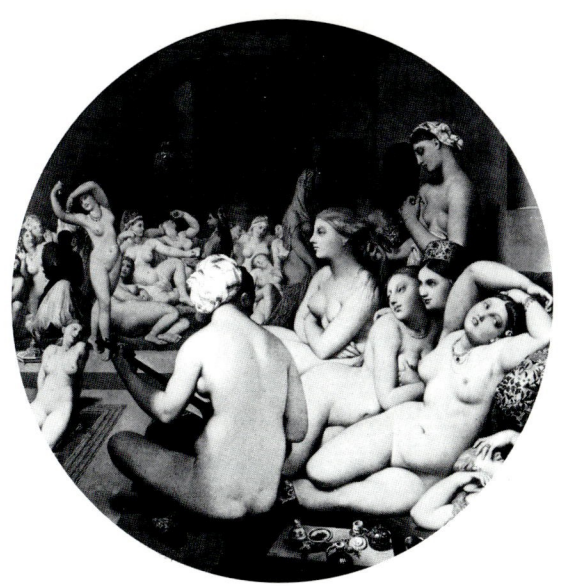

Albrecht Dürer was one of the first to introduce realism into his studies of the nude, as in the figure at the right of this drawing of women bathing (above left). The bath, became a favourite subject in art, of which Ingres (above) took full advantage. Other suitable subjects were incidents from classical literature, exemplified by Cornelis van Haarlem's *Marriage of Peleus and Thetis* (below left). And even in the Dublin Metropolitan School of Art, by the end of the Victorian era, the study of the live nude was considered a suitable subject for both male and female art students (below).

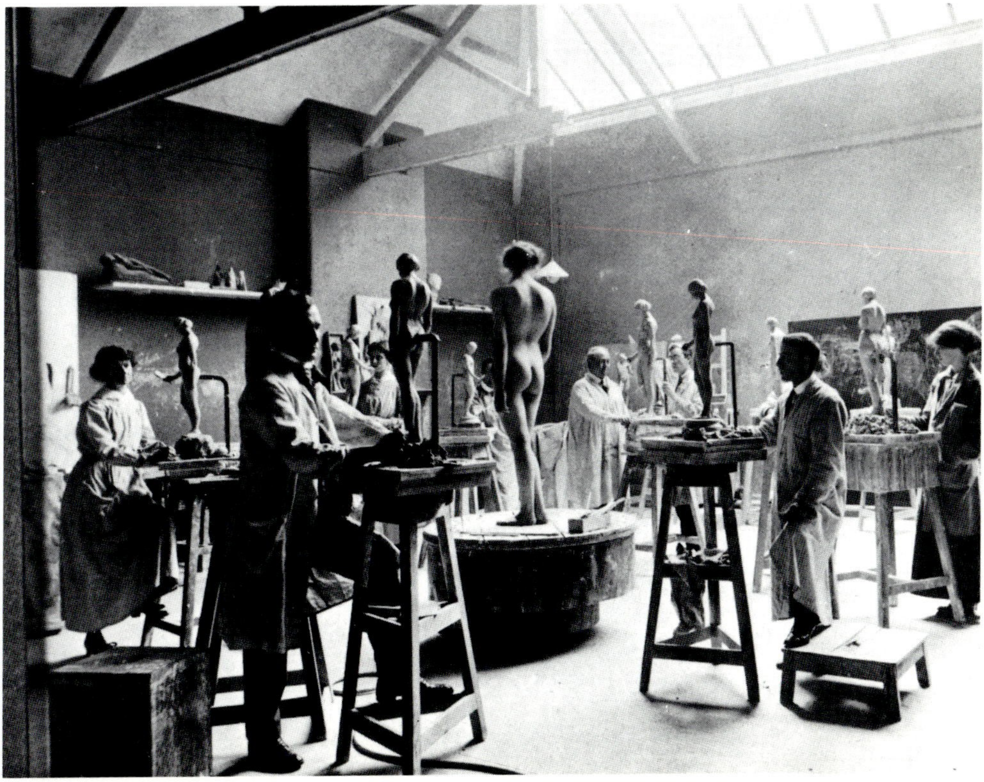

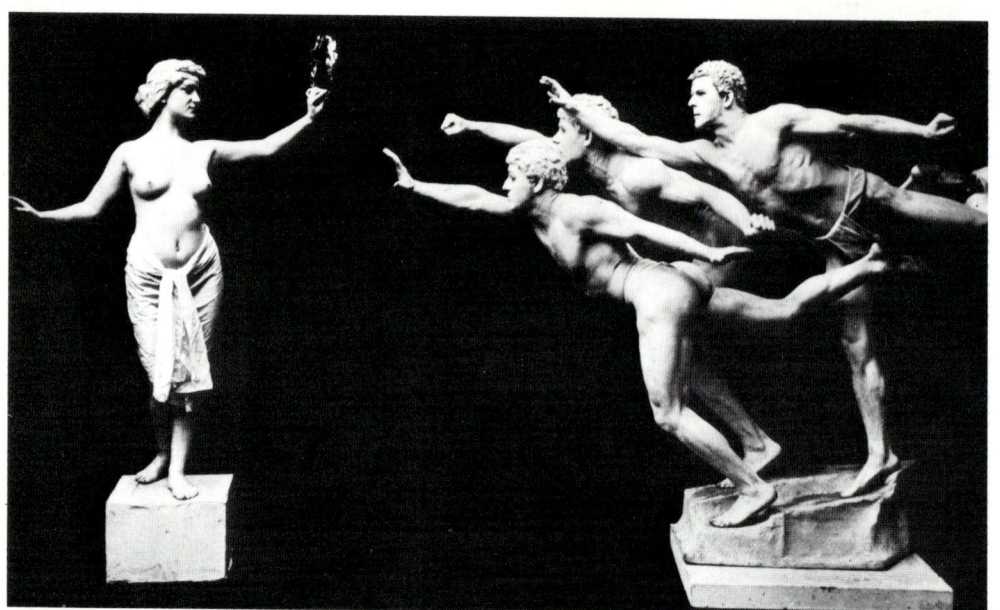

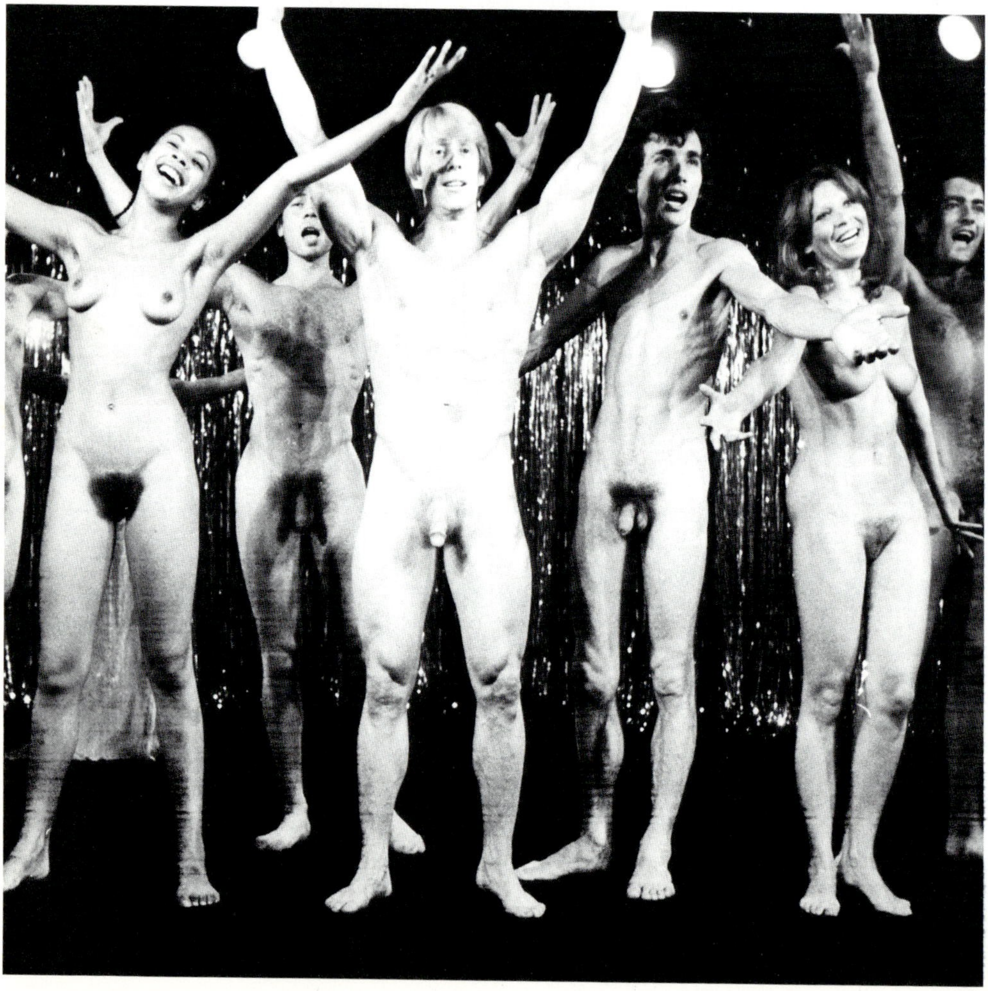

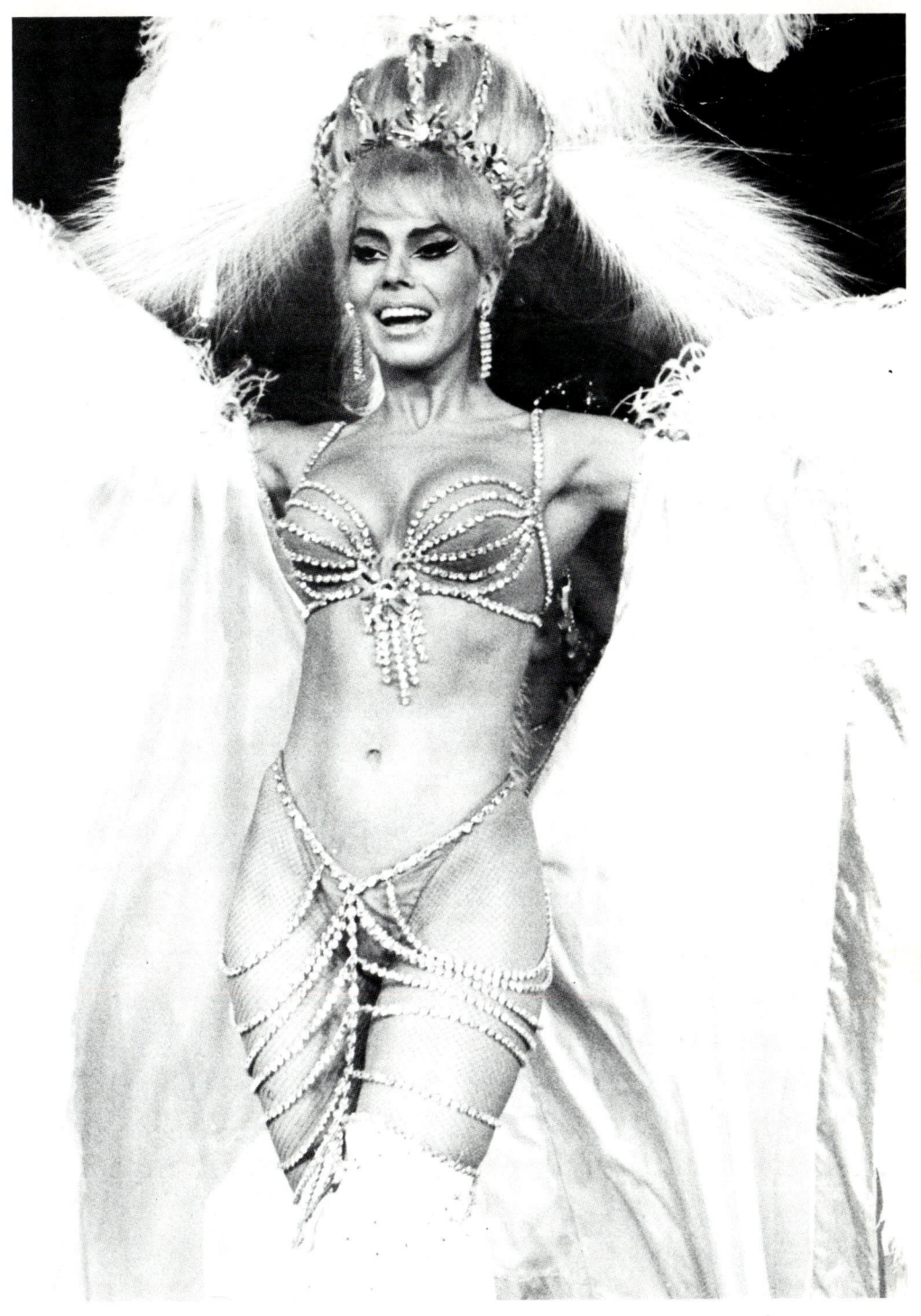

Nudity on the stage has a very ancient history, and it has consistently defied the prevailing morality. Even the Victorians permitted the famous 'poses plastiques' (above left). The English production of *Oh Calcutta!* (below left) celebrated the abolition of stage censorship; but more conventional stage presentations combine total or near-nudity with the most exotic costumes imaginable (above).

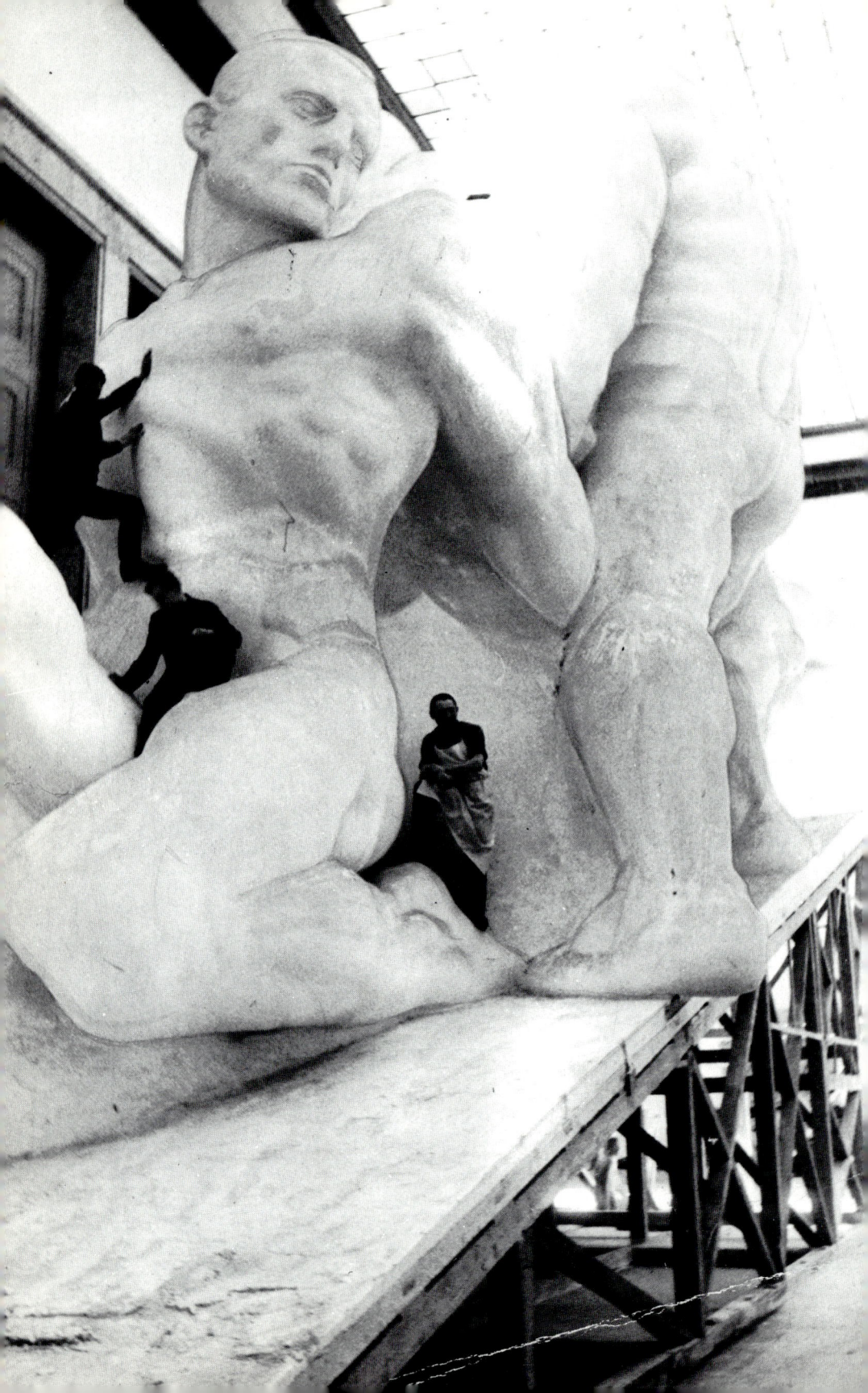

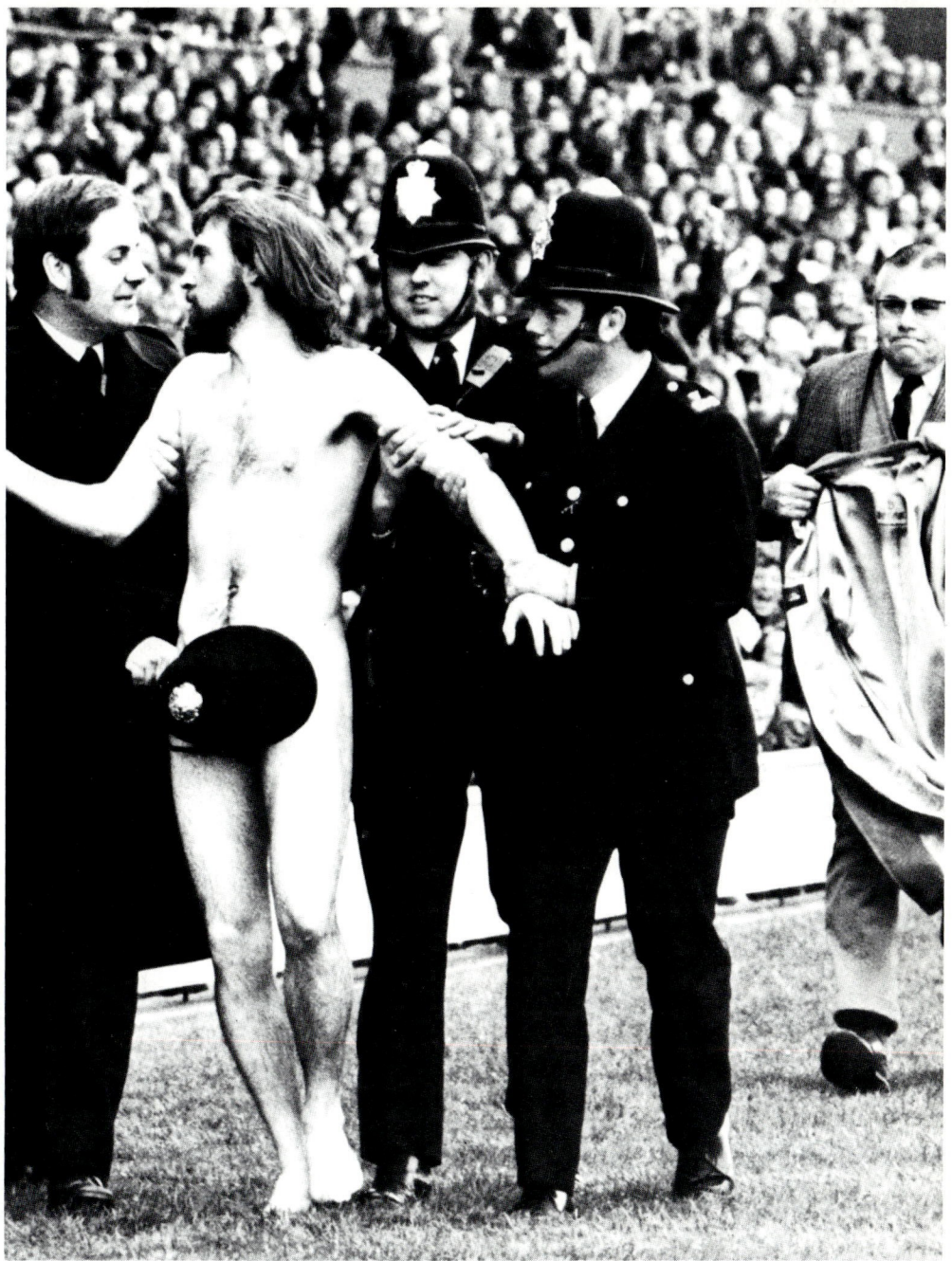

Throughout all the ups and downs of conventional attitudes to nakedness in art, the nude figure, male or female, has remained acceptable in public statuary, often celebrating martial triumph. These vast figures, now demolished (left), were commissioned by the Nazis in anticipation of their ultimate victory in the Second World War. The appearance of 'streakers' at football or cricket matches, however (above), is not considered acceptable.

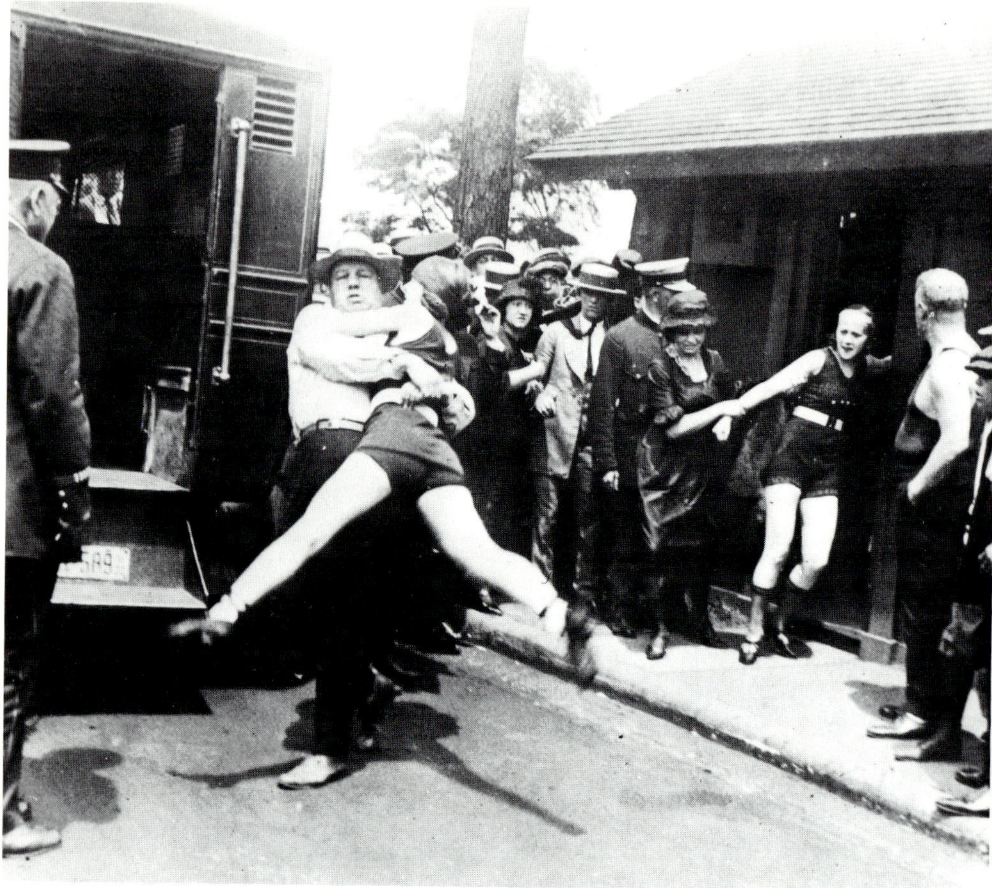

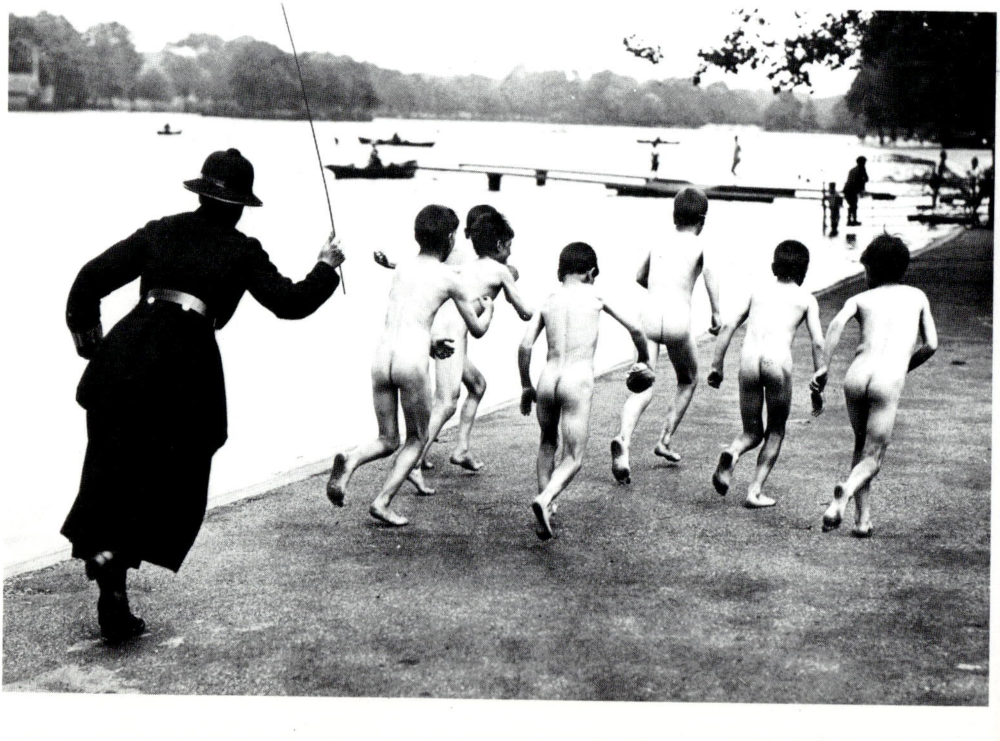

Until well into the nineteenth century, nude bathing contrived to escape the strictures of popular moralists. 'A Back-Side and Front View of a Modern Fine Lady or Swimming Venus' (right) could provide 'Summer Amusement at Margate' (below) in the eighteenth century. But attitudes changed. Girl swimmers were arrested in Boston in 1909 (left) for wearing a man's bathing suit which exposed the legs and arms; and even little boys in London's Serpentine were not immune from the wrath of a well-armed policewoman (below left).

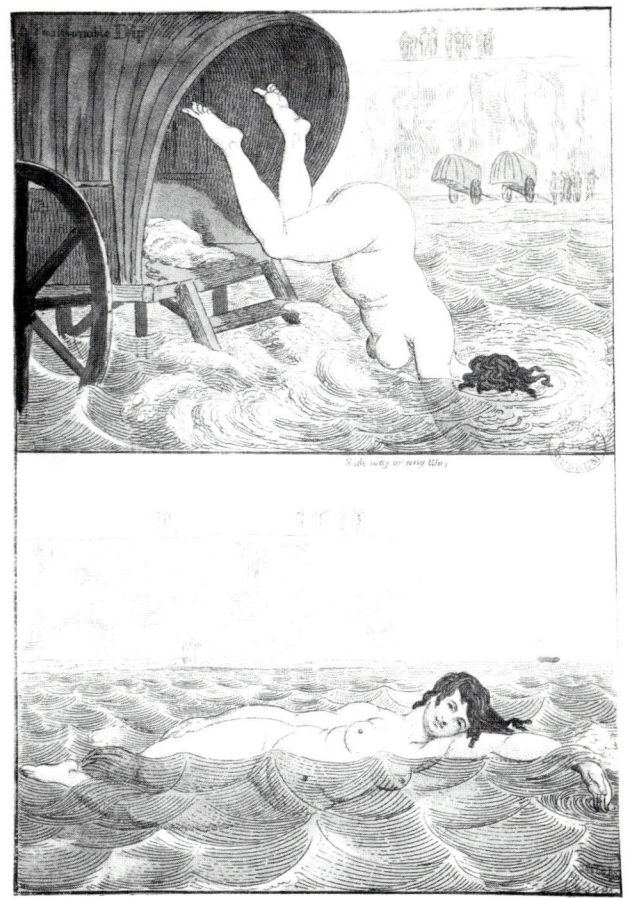

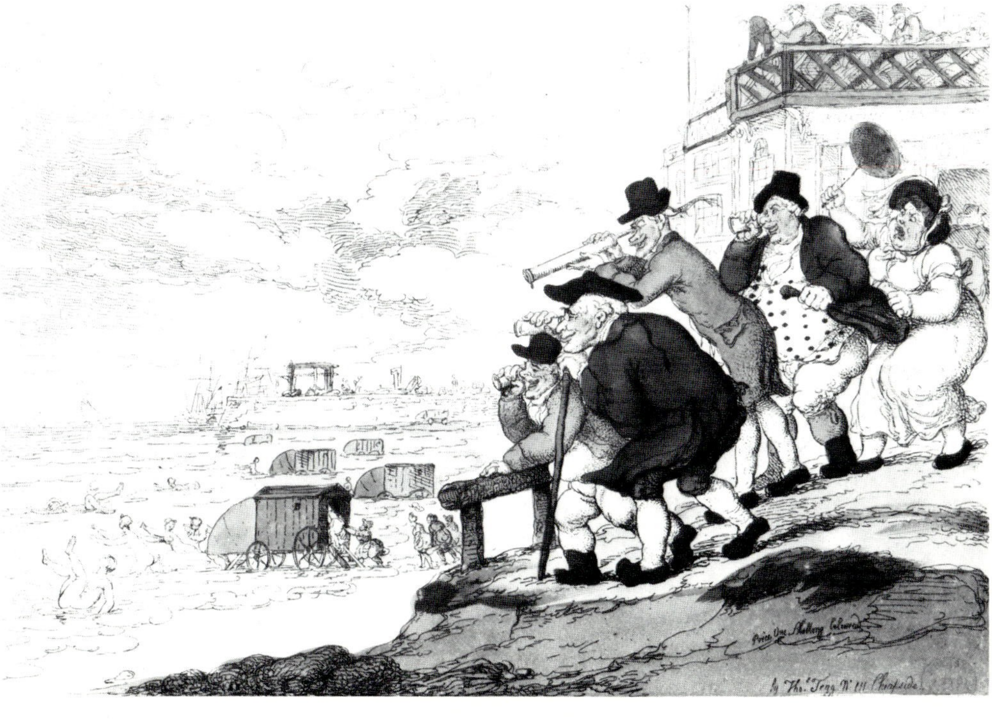

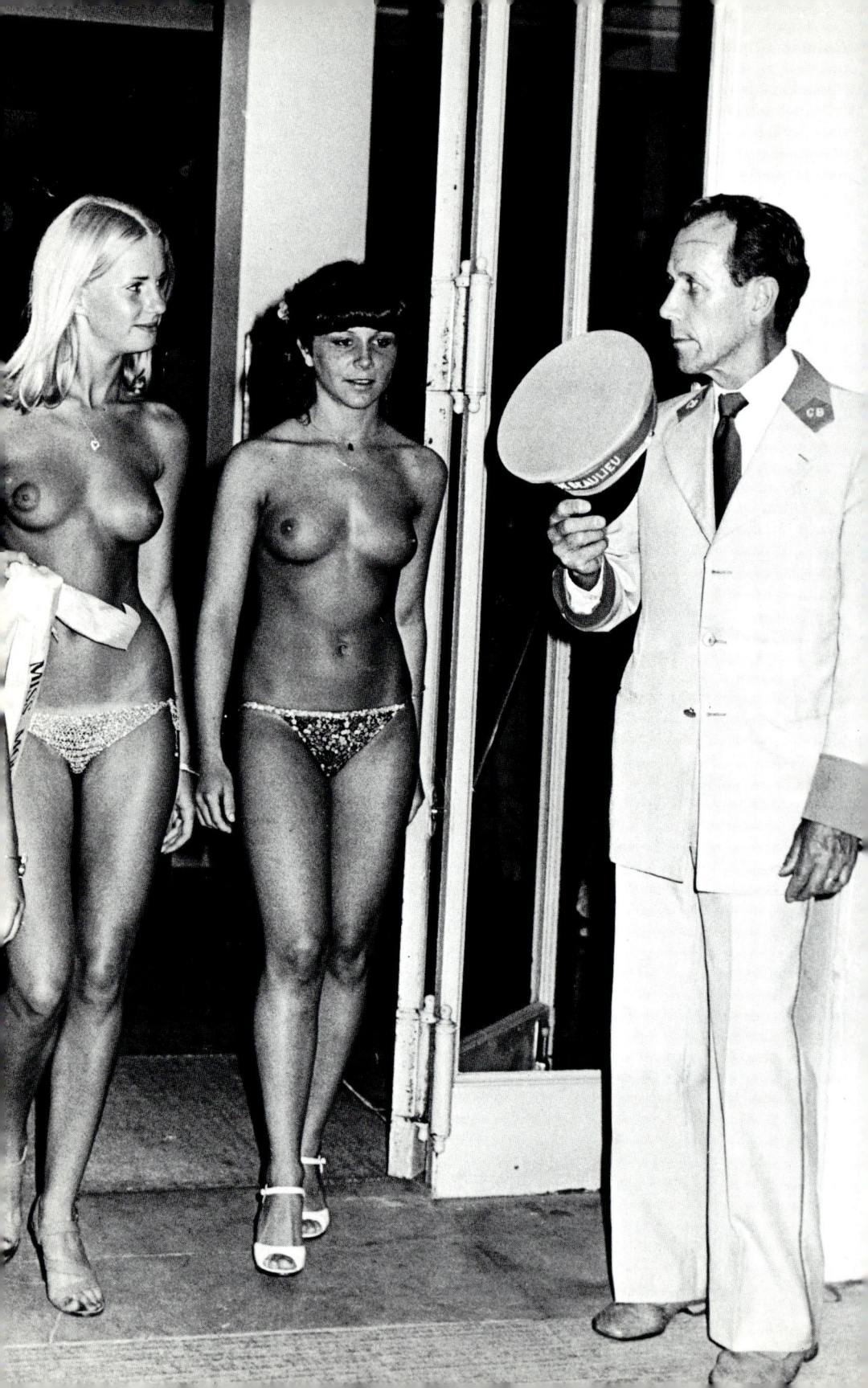

Attitudes to beach nudity have relaxed markedly in recent years. The 'monokini' (left) is acceptable wear not only on the beaches but in the hotels of the Côte d'Azur; and along the coasts of France and Yugoslavia (right) whole resorts have been built where total nudity is the norm. Yet as recently as 1955, *Sunbathing Annual*, which promised 'intimate glimpses of nudists' private lives', thought it necessary to obliterate all suggestion of sexuality from its pictures (below).

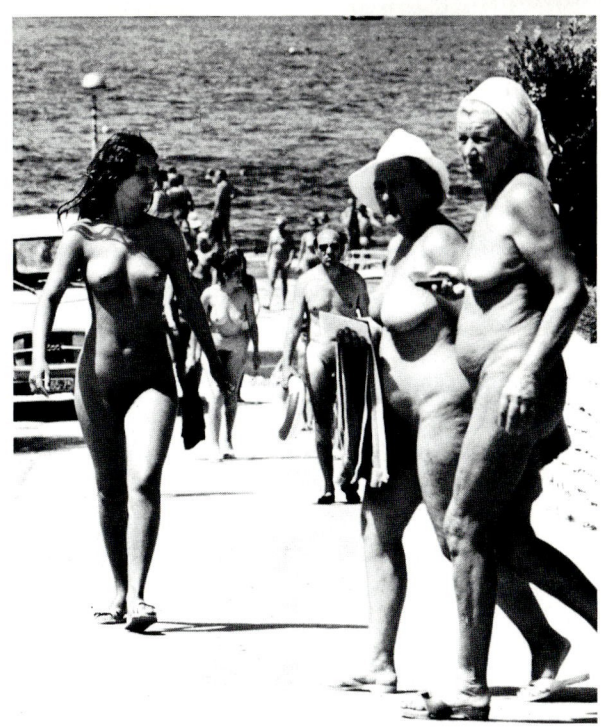

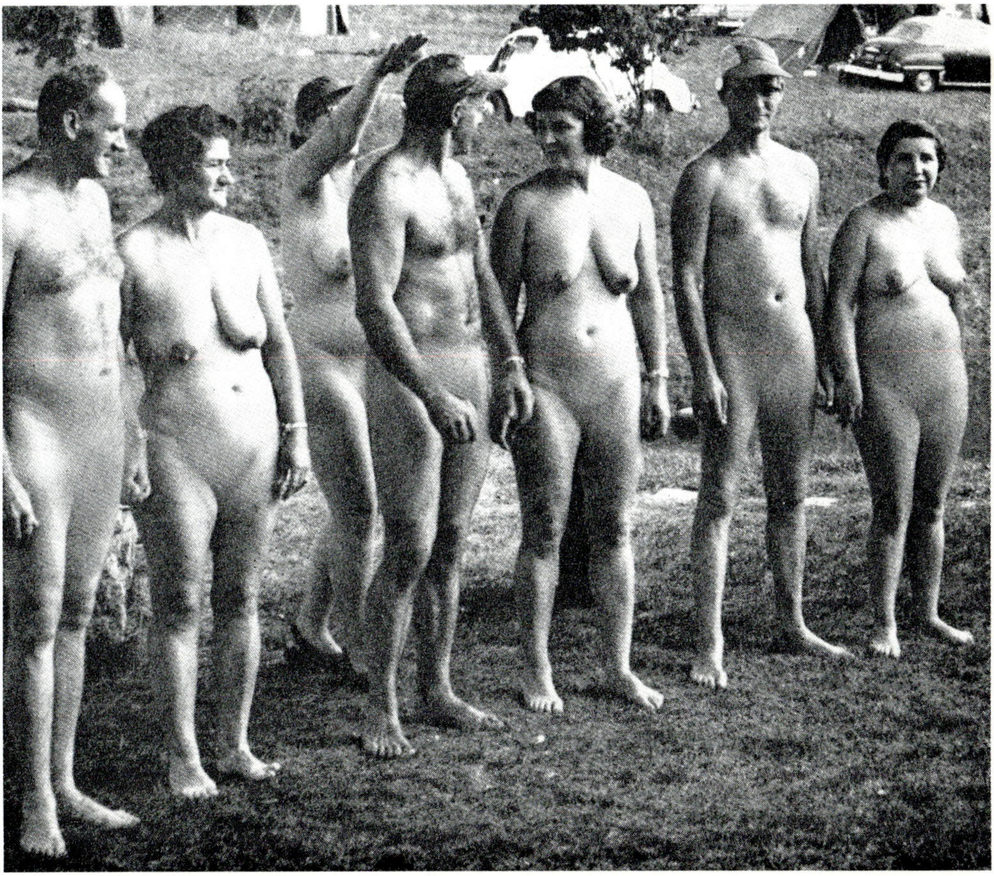

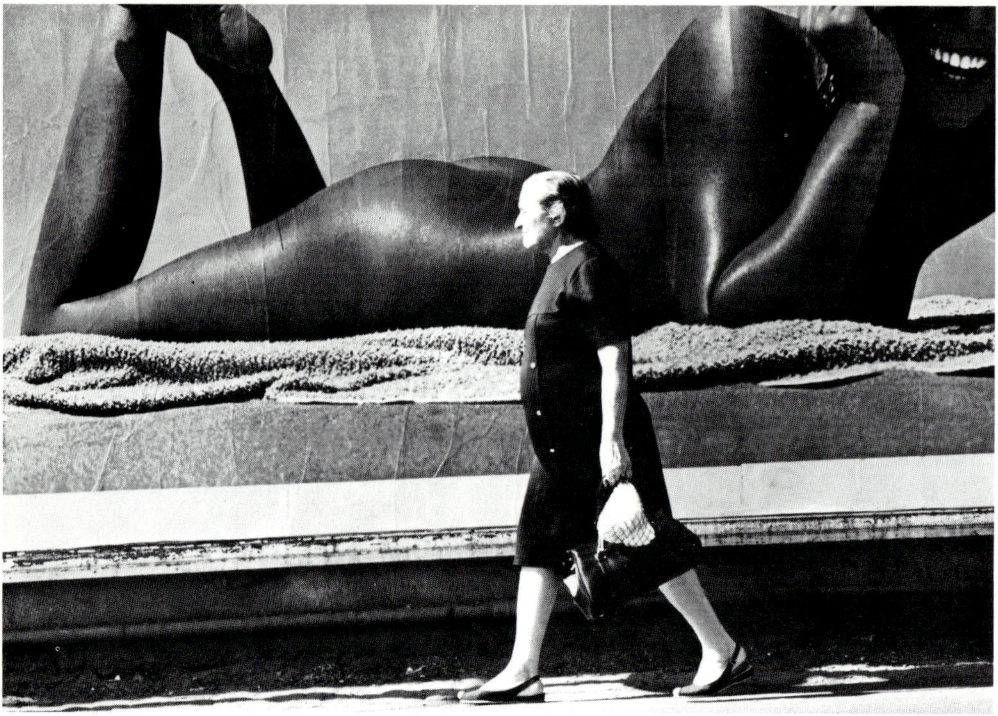

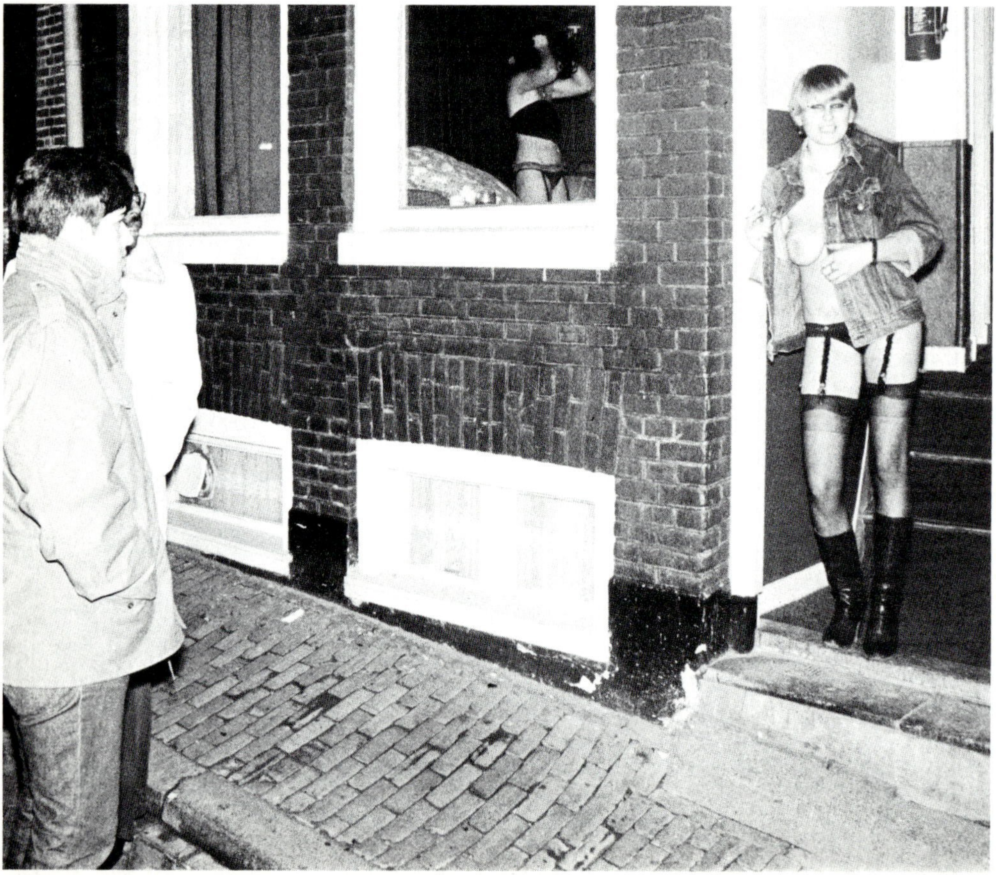

The display of the female body derives from repressed sexuality and the voyeuristic impulse. In public it may be acceptable or unacceptable: passers-by scarcely give a second glance to a vast advertisement for suntan oil (left); but the prostitute displaying her wares in an Amsterdam doorway (below left) attracts considerable prurient interest. The appeal of the pin-up is universal, but it can take many forms, from the aggressively 'respectable' but lavishly exposed image put forward by Jayne Mansfield (below) to the pointedly perverse but concealed anatomy of a Pirelli calendar (right).

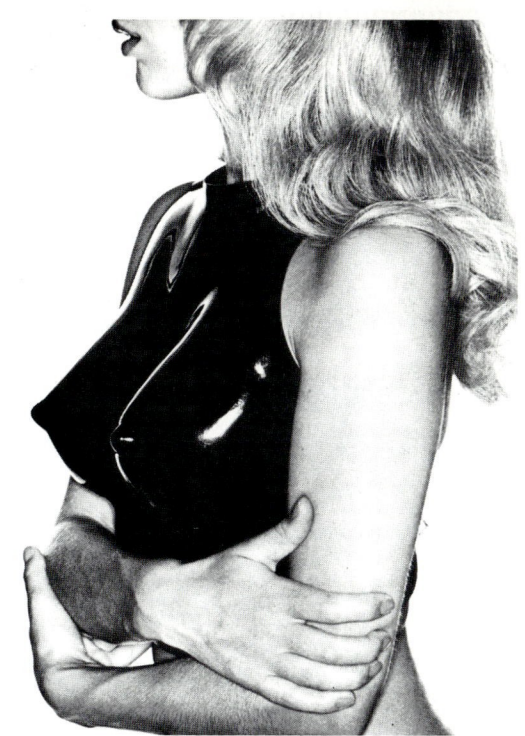

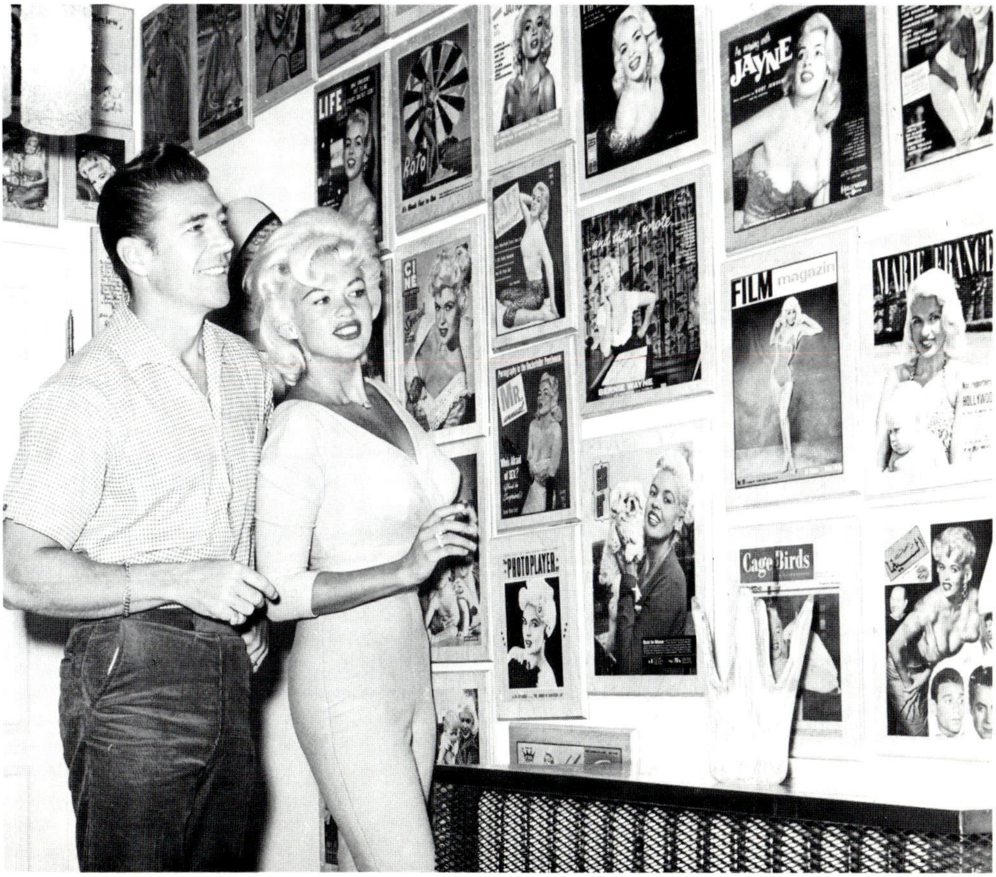

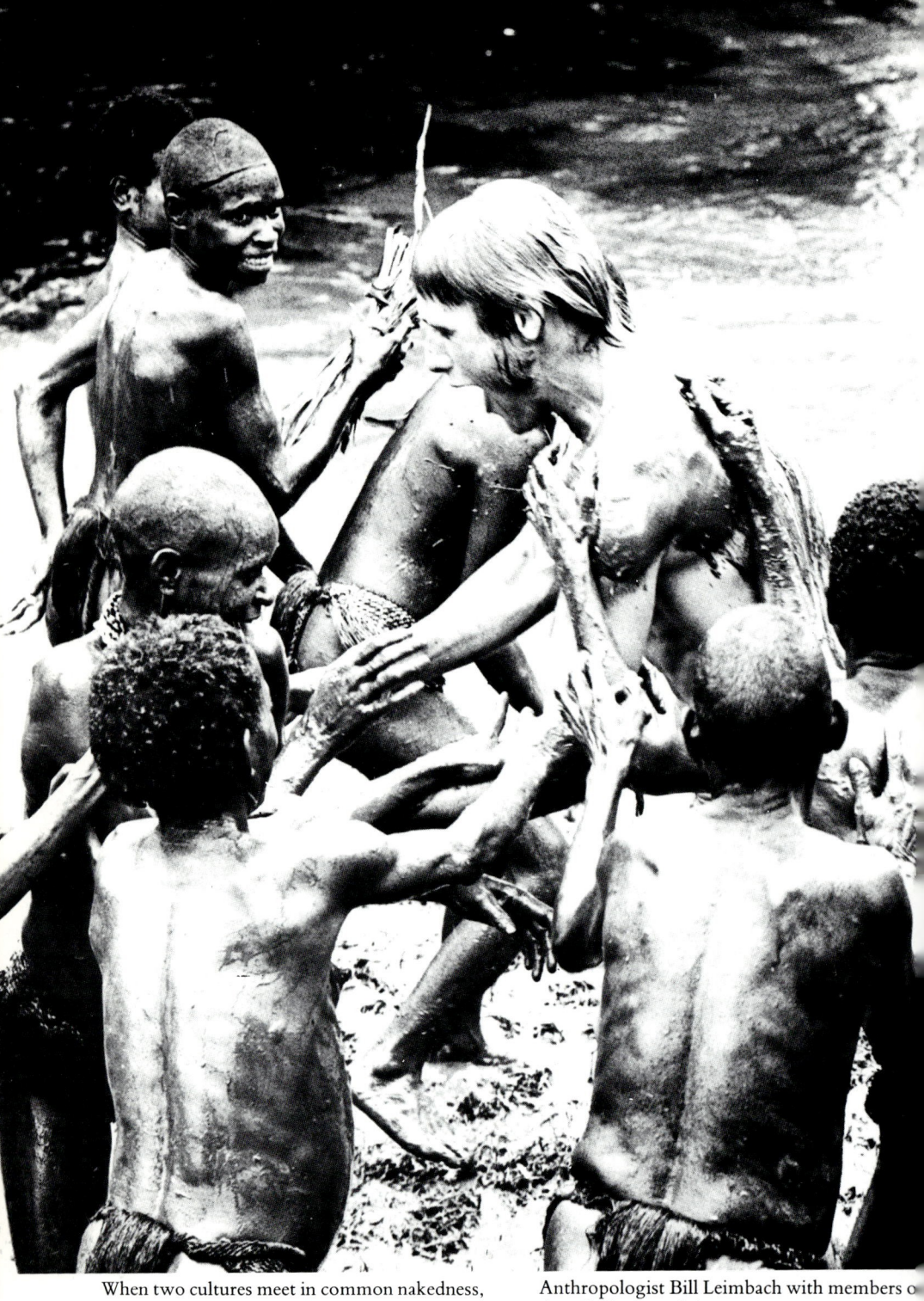

When two cultures meet in common nakedness, which is the observed and which is the observer?

Anthropologist Bill Leimbach with members of the tribe he is studying.

island all work stopped and the whole population turned out to welcome 'the players'. And they were true players who were adept at 'dancing, singing, wrestling ... spear-fighting ... and plays of different kinds'. After a kind of religious prologue, for example 'a description of the two principles of life, of the god Taaroa and how he united himself with matter, and the creation of the universe, gods, elements, spirits, plants and other products of the earth', the company would concentrate on the more diversionary side of their programme. The plays performed, according to Daniellson, span virtually the complete range to be found in the West End at the time of writing. The actors and actresses offered historical dramas, political sketches and songs 'containing extremely pointed references to current events', pure comic turns and pantomimes and nude dances. They also included one other element, which had both a mystical and an entertainment value for the audience, and which can only be found in the modern theatre in simulation – exhibitions of sexual intercourse. We have a description of such a scene by a no less scrupulous observer than Captain James Cook: 'A young man, nearly six feet high, performed the rites of Venus with a little girl about eleven or twelve years of age, before several of our people, and a great number of the natives, without the least sense of its being indecent or improper, but, as appeared, in perfect conformity to the custom of the place. Among the spectators were several women of superior rank, who may properly be said to have assisted at the ceremony; for they gave instructions to the girl how to perform her part, which, young as she was, she did not seem much to stand in need of.'

This description elicited from Voltaire in France the comment: 'It can be affirmed that the inhabitants of Tahiti have preserved the oldest religion on earth in all its purity.' What Voltaire failed to mention was that what the crew of *The Endeavour* had observed was also the oldest theatrical performance on earth in all its purity. It has been remarked before that the act of sex is itself a miniature model of a play. According to Peter Webb in *The Erotic Arts*, plays manifest 'a wide variety of plot-constructions leading in every case to a similar variety of climaxes'. He quotes the American dramatist Robert Anderson saying: 'Comedy is like petting: it's fun and no one gets hurt. A serious play is more like intercourse: if you don't have an orgasm, you end up frustrated.' It is interesting that the same word 'climax' is used to describe the end of a play and of an act of sex, and Aristotle's description of the purpose of tragedy as *catharsis*, the purging of the mind of pity and terror, has an obvious parallel in sexual orgasm.

As regards Western civilization, the theatre proper starts with the Greeks. It came, inevitably, from religious roots, the first theatres being places of worship with tiers of spectators surrounding an altar. Gradually the altar became a stage and the spectators, housed in vast outdoor amphitheatres, a true audience. This early Greek theatre remained close to its religious roots, but already the split between what might be called 'sublimated' theatre, that which has distanced itself from its erotic base, and bawdy theatre had begun to manifest itself. The Greeks were in no sense puritanical about sex. Their versions of the orgiastic dance took place in city festivals in honour of Dionysus where gigantic models of the phallus were carried through the streets and general debauchery accompanied the celebrations. In wealthy Athenian homes obscene playlets were performed, often by slaves, for the delight of the guests. But in the great theatres of Greece, drama had already diversified into serious theatre, which in this context meant tragedy, and the satyr plays, which were lewd knockabouts. This division has remained ever since and both components have proved equally durable. In the West End of London at the present day audiences are watching theatrical displays varying from simulated, and probably in very secret locations, actual, sexual intercourse through to grand drama which, superficially at least, has little to do with the naked human body.

> God knows what will follow on stage if *Oh! Calcutta!* can get away
> with criminal acts of corruption and depravity . . . Such a crime
> against human dignity and values . . . I no longer wish to belong to
> a society which causes me so much pain by allowing the dear
> humanity I cherish to be openly and savagely abused.

These are the words of David Holbrook, the moralist and author, writing in *The Times* in 1970 on the occasion of the transfer of the now-celebrated erotic review from New York to London. Two reflections are engendered. The first is that in an age which has included extermination camps in Germany, the Gulug Archipelago in Russia, the frying of whole cities with nuclear weapons; 'dear humanity' has been more 'openly and savagely abused' than by a daring stage show. As a corollary, it seems Mr Holbrook has based his desired withdrawal from our culture on grounds that themselves reflect a gross perversion of values. But the second consideration is the one germane to this chapter. *Oh! Calcutta!* is a paradigm, and quite a mild one, of voyeuristic sexual entertainments which are endemic to clothed and repressed societies. For thousands of years the moralists of the world have been denouncing and, when in power, attempting to suppress, analogous responses to erotic frustration. They might just as well fulminate against breathing. In fact, it is the concealment and the repression that constitute the disease. Displays like *Oh! Calcutta!* are merely the symptom and closing them down has no more effect on the patient than painting out the spots would have on an infectious disease.

Needless to say, the history of such displays is very similar to the history of those of the other manifestations of sexuality we have considered: repression and re-emergence. The Greek and Roman theatre, especially the private theatre conducted in the homes of the rich, was prodigal of playlets and sketches, often based on the scandalous doings of the gods. In the Middle Ages, theatre in Europe was almost exclusively restricted to miracle and mystery plays, based on scripture. But here too, an element of body display often appeared. Adam and Eve in the garden of Eden supplied a good pretext and were often represented nude or in what we would call body-stockings. Marc de Montifoaux describes a bawdy incident that occurred during a village performance of a Good Friday mystery play. A handsome young man, virtually naked, was attached to a cross in order to represent Christ. Before him, three of the prettiest girls in town were on their knees with lightly-covered bosoms, representing the three Marys, whereupon 'a very comic and profane incident' occurred.

The modern theatre has its origins in the sixteenth century, at which time an impresario called Galosi opened a theatre in Paris which 'started with erotic playlets but the exhibition of nakedness soon lost its naive character and became frankly obscene'. At the time of the French Revolution, the authorities, like other reforming bodies before and since, hoped to use the theatre as a means of propagating right thinking and spreading social education. At the great Paris theatres, the *Opéra* and the *Comédie Française*, ennobling art was the order of the day. But in the numerous small theatres the old licentiousness continued. Proudhon, an ideologist of the later revolution of 1848, was especially incensed about a small theatre at the Palais Royal which had an intriguing sign outside which invitingly proclaimed 'Enter, Gentlemen, you will see inside the great ballet of the savages'. Proudhon felt it his guardian's duty to investigate and found that inside 'you see a pretend savage and his wife, both of them naked and who, in the presence of the spectators, deliver themselves up to the most secret mysteries of nature'.

Although it is technically far easier to suppress stage nudity than to eliminate prostitution, finding a rationale for doing so has proved more testing for authorities. This is because it has been virtually an aesthetic axiom in the West since Greek civilization that the human body is the most beautiful thing in the universe. How then can one justify the denial of this presumably exalting spectacle to the populace? The supposed divine proportions and line of the body have regularly provided an argument by which nudity or near-nudity has made its way back to the stage. The Victorians were very censorious of impropriety but even they were compelled to permit the famous 'poses plastiques'. These were still representations by living men and women (actors and actresses would be a ludicrous designation in such a context) of simulated sculptural scenes or copies of actual sculptured groups. This device enabled respectable people to enthuse about the 'artistic value' of the spectacle while actually gratifying their voyeuristic urge. As recently as the fifties in London, at the Windmill Theatre, although the pretence of being 'living statues' had been abandoned, the girls were only allowed to be totally naked if they were motionless. The popular phrase 'if it moves its rude' accurately expressed the official attitude. By the seventies, we reached the stage of *Oh! Calcutta!*, a show which features some quite pretty nude dancing, some mildly offensive, schoolboyish, rude dialogue and a certain amount of simulated copulation between members of an authentically naked cast. I personally found one or two of the sketches amusing, some of the dancing attractive, and quite a lot of the show offensive – but offensive *because* is represented the prurience indissociable from repression, rather than because it was a genuine escape from it.

It has been left to the Americans, a traditionally pragmatic people, to devise what is probably the exact expression of the hunger for the lost body in a repressed culture: the strip-tease. Basically, this is simply the public removal of her clothes by a more-or-less attractive woman. Since this operation would be too brief to be commercially justifiable, it is padded with a little movement, even a few dance-steps, possibly some singing or dialogue, and it may be incorporated in a little sketch. In England recently there was a vogue for male strippers, who performed before clamourous and unruly female audiences, which suggests that when women are not impeded by an imposed image of how they should behave they seek visual body gratification just as men do.

Seymour Fisher, in his excellent *Body Consciousness* suggests that the impulse to see a strip-tease expresses more than erotic frustration and that, in a clothed society, a fundamental anxiety as to the continued existence of the body uneasily subsists in all of us. Watching someone undress, and seeing their body emerge intact from its ordeal by clothing, reassures us that the natural order is still operational.

Witkowski and Nass, writing in 1909, state:

> The theatre has always been and will always be the animated representation of life . . . We go to the theatre to hear people speak of love, of ethereal love, of lawful or unlawful love, of licentious love, what does it matter?

Sixty years later, Desmond Morris in *The Naked Ape* restated this truth at greater length and with at least an approach to supplying a scientific explanation of the fascination:

> Although the powerful sexual imprinting keeps the mated pair together, it does not eliminate their interest in outside sexual activities. If outside matings conflict too strongly with the pair-bond, then some less harmful substitute for them has to be found. The solution has been voyeurism, using the term in its broadest sense, and this is employed on an enormous scale. In the strict sense voyeurism means obtaining sexual excitement from watching other individuals copulating, but it can logically be broadened out to include any non-participatory interest in any sexual activity. Almost the entire population indulges in this. They watch it, they read about it, they listen to it. The vast bulk of all television, radio, cinema, theatre and fiction-writing is concerned with satisfying this demand.

But, of course, the satisfactions of the voyeuristic impulse provided by the media are themselves sublimated and synthetic. They are no real substitute for living in an unconcealed society where the body and its functions are part of the normal environment. Most people in civilized communities manage to satisfy their instinctual desire for 'carnal knowledge' with the available surrogates, including pornography, as well as the outlets, deliberate or inadvertent, that even a repressed society cannot totally eliminate. But there are important minorities at either end of the spectrum who can be conveniently dubbed ascetics and perverts. The ascetics are those who succeed in converting all or almost all of their erotic drive into 'cultural' activity. They constitute a remarkable class, unknown to primitive societies, which includes great benefactors who have given the world some of its loftiest thought and art, but also embraces demonic individuals whose frustrated sexuality results in misanthropy. The perverts, a term I use here in a purely classificatory sense, are those who, for one reason or another, are not satisfied with the socially approved outlets for their impulse to see and to be seen. They are called, in the language of psychoanalysis, voyeurs and exhibitionists. It is remarkable that nowhere in the history of psychoanalytic thought (and since such claims are always booby-traps, I had better immediately add insofar as I have ever seen) is there any suggestion that the fundamental perversion, to which many, if not all, particular perversions are essentially responses, is the concealment of the body that has resulted from the universal adoption of clothes. From this perspective, calling voyeurism and exhibitionism 'perversions' is like calling the hungry man's obsessive concern with food perversion. These 'perversions' are, in my opinion, simply assertions of instinctual imperatives, manifesting themselves in ways that a clothed society has outlawed.

Concerning the prevalent, but muffled, voyeuristic acitivity of our species, Desmond Morris concludes:

> It is comparatively harmless and may actually help . . . because it satisfies to some extent the persistent demands of our sexual curiosity without involving the individuals concerned in new potential mateship relationships that could threaten the pair-bond.

This is woefully inadequate. The erotic drive or instinct is of such power and pervasiveness throughout human culture that our very survival on this planet may well depend on what we make of it. To suggest that the preservation of 'pair-bond' 'mateship' by means of surrogate voyeurism may help, when the history of clothed civilization indicates that murderous frustration characterizes our culture, is a disservice to the race. Admittedly, connections are not linear, and may not even be traceable, but what we do with our instincts and what we do with our weapons are undoubtedly connected. The sexual repression that is most obviously and pervasively expressed by concealing clothing is one of the threats to our future.

BACK TO EDEN

In 1979, a Bournemouth councillor remarked (and *The Observer* reprinted in its 'Sayings of the Week' column), 'Naturists would pollute the beach.' Her indignation had been provoked by a proposal that Brighton, and other English seaside resorts, should initiate official 'naturist beaches'.

Now naked sea-bathers on the English coast would be no new thing. As a columnist in the *Evening Standard* said, 'The Brighton fathers are merely resurrecting a custom which was common on our beaches throughout most of history and ending a ban which has only a century of tradition behind it.' People have bathed naked in the sea since people started to bathe at all.

But the polluting hordes fearfully awaited at Brighton were not just people coming to bathe without absurdly first putting on the required garments, but 'naturists'. What distinguishes a 'naturist' from any kid peeling off his togs, kicking away his shoes and running bare-ass into the briny? The difference is not easy to define, but essentially a 'naturist' is someone who believes in the beneficial properties of nakedness which can be spiritual and psychological as well as physical, rather than someone who considers nakedness expedient, convenient or simply fun, or who practises it intermittently like, say, the Doukhobors, as part of a broader pattern of ideas. While having precursors, naturism mainly belongs to the twentieth century. It is a thriving and expanding movement and has already taken on some of the properties of a sub-culture.

Individuals have throughout the ages extolled the beneficial properties of nakedness. Even in puritanical (as it was until quite recently)

America, men like Benjamin Franklin and Thoreau have praised, and occasionally practised in a domestic context, nakedness. But it was left to Senancour in *De l'Amour considéré dans les lois réelles et dans les formes sociales de l'union des deux sexes*, first published in 1805, to provide a manifesto for the naturist movement.

> Let us suppose a country in which at certain general festivals the women should be absolutely free to be nearly or even quite naked. Swimming, waltzing, walking, those who thought good to do so might remain unclothed in the presence of men ... Such nakedness would demand corresponding institutions, strong and simple, and a great respect for those conventions which belong to all times.

If the scope of his remarks were extended to include both sexes, and a few remarks as to the positive value of nakedness were added, this declaration would be quite suitable for a modern naturist.

At the heart of the twentieth-century naturist movement is the idea of health. This is not surprising since the progenitors most often mentioned by virtually all authorities are doctors.

A medical movement involving sun-bathing came about in the early part of this century as a reaction to traditional methods of treatment such as the loathsome practise of enfeebling already weak patients by bleeding them with leeches or suction. It was also an acknowledgement of new medical insight, spearheaded by the pathogenic discovers of Pasteur, which suggested that fresh air and hygiene might be of more value in the recovery of health than the medicines then available. This movement represented a reaction to the stuffy, enclosed, unwholesome environment that had prevailed in Europe for centuries reaching its apogee in Victorian times. It went hand in hand with the emergence of new concepts in regard to personal hygiene and domestic and civic sanitation. An important aspect of this movement was a new critical attitude to the whole matter of clothing. It was realized that fashion had almost totally ignored the physiological requirements of the body and that many common garments were insanitary, often constituting virtual pastures for parasites, while others actually distorted the body and impaired its functions. Once critical attention had been directed towards clothing and 'dress reform' was being widely debated it was only a short step to asking whether the absence of clothing might not prove to be the healthiest 'garment' of all.

The medical and ideological basis for naturism was established before the First World War mainly in Germany, and during the twenties nudism was largely confined to Germany. Visitors from America and various European countries, however, carried reports of the wonders of nudism back to their home countries and the first steps were taken towards the establishment of centres in other parts of the world. In Scandinavia and Russia, where nude bathing was a traditional part of life, the tidings caused little stir and less activity, but in England, America and France the campaign of official hostility and media derision, which still continues, began. Many people, who have no knowledge of nudism, assume that it is associated with extreme political views. Koch's socialist nudist movement in Germany represented the closest official affiliation of the movement with politics. There is no connection, or only a negative one, between nudism and the Nazis since Hitler banned the movement in Germany with the words, 'The total exposure of the human body is undignified as well as an error of taste.' Thus, from the Hitler period onwards, the focus of nudism shifted from Germany to America and England. In England, nudism was associated with 'progressive' rather than political movements. All through the thirties nudism spread slowly in America, France and England, although it reached nothing like the dimensions it had achieved in Germany in the twenties.

The chief features of nudism since the Second World War have been its steady progress and its tendency to establish itself in climatically suitable places. In Europe, the logical region for the practice is around the Mediterranean. From Perpignan to Dalmatia there are now substantial nudist establishments and 'topless' swimming is becoming the norm even in Portugal. Whatever the success of those who seek to establish a nudist beach at Brighton, the English Channel is unlikely to draw the same crowds as the mild to sub-tropical Mediterranean.

What are the claims made for nudism and how far have they been proved valid? Before embarking on personal, and hence subjective, experiences and estimates I will try to look objectively at some reports of others. It is important to say initially that very little serious scientific research into the alleged benefits has ever been done. Nudism has been from its inception, and largely remains, a polemical battlefield between fervent advocates and passionate antagonists. The dispatches from this war-zone are unreliable, but they are all we have.

In the first place, what of the claims made as regards physical benefits? In the early days, these were often absurdly excessive. Thus Langdon-Davies in his book *The Future of Nakedness* (1929) describes a 'before' photograph from Rollier's work *Heliotherapy*. The picture shows an unfortunate small boy: 'the knees are larger than the hips, the elbow larger than the shoulder, the feet have become transformed into shapeless sores, the stomach is a swollen bag of poison, the hands are a supporating mass of filth . . .' But 'after many months of the cure' the same boy is revealed 'making a hayrick, lifting a heavy stone' and in every way a vigourous specimen. Langdon-Davies asks:

> What has produced this miracle? He has been fed properly, rested properly, made to sleep, but, far more important than this, Dr Rollier has taken off his clothes . . . the sun and the air have rushed in and killed the loathsome enemy in his tissues . . .

The trouble here, of course, is that it is impossible to determine which benefits derived from the nakedness. Probably few modern doctors would be disposed to believe that the boy's recovery would have been very different if he had worn a vest and trunks but otherwise received the same wholesome treatment.

The truth is that, in spite of quite convincing testimony that wearing wet bathing suits for long periods of time can result in rheumatic complaints, there is little or no hard evidence to prove that nudism is physically beneficial. Nudists certainly tend to be healthy people but this is just as likely to be because the movement attracts those who look after their bodies and take a pride in their physical well-being, as because it promotes health. Still, even the movement's most articulate opponents have rarely claimed that nudism is actually harmful to health. The balance of probability is on the side of the nudists.

Another strong line of advocacy by nudists has been the moral one. Nudists have always claimed that common nudity between the sexes *decreases* sexual tension and harmonizes intersexual relationships. They maintain that a far higher degree of sexual morality prevails in nudist camps than elsewhere, and that all unwholesome curiosity is dissipated. They emphasize that nudity provides children with the only natural way of becoming familiar with the basic facts of sexual physiology and enables them to grow up without the tormenting curiosity and hole-in-corner experimentation which characterize childhood in clothed societies. A portion of this advocacy undoubtedly stems from propagandist motives. To the non-initiate the idea of many naked men and women living together inevitably conjures up the idea of licence and even orgy. In America, early nudist establishments were dubbed by the tabloid press 'love-colonies'. In fact, nudist establishments have been essentially family-oriented. Even today it is difficult for single males to obtain access to them. The claims of high moral values have undoubtedly been justified. Traditionally, a kind of puritanism has governed the regulation of nudist establishments and it is virtually certain that orthodox sexual morality has been higher inside nudist establishments than in the world at large. But this may prove to have been a phenomenon required for initial acceptance rather than an inherent part of the concept of nudism. Finally, it is almost certainly true that children benefit. Many people will recall from their own childhoods, and literary accounts amply confirm, that sexual curiosity can be a great burden. Children who have had regular experience of nudism are undoubtedly less susceptible to this misery.

There have, in fact, been very few serious psychological or sociological studies of nudism. One of the few psychoanalysts who visited a nudist camp, not as an enthusiast but as an investigator, submitted his report under initials only. His anonymity parallels that of many nudists who, to this day, take great care that friends and neighbours do not learn of their pastime. The report dates from 1939 and concerns experiences in an American establishment. In part, it says:

> I think one effect of social nudism is to battle against what I may call the age-old psychological enemy of modern mankind – the isolation of sex. If you were in psychotherapy, you would see very clearly that at the bottom of most nervous disorders is a very distorted and very painful attitude towards the other sex. In strong language, you can almost say that for many men women are mostly a big vagina with something attached to it, or a big trap in which they can fall and be swallowed. Men are to many women just aggressive penises with something behind. It is unbelievable how few people are really able to conceive of a member of the other sex as another human being ... one of the automatic effects of social nudism is that the sexual organs are *reintegrated* [his italics] into the human body ...

Essentially, human beings in a habitually clothed society consist of naked, talking heads and concealed genitals. The imagination is perpetually striving to unify these two manifestations of almost irreconcilable realities. The 'intelligent', verbalizing head is the expression of culture, civilization, social life, work and war. The hidden genitals are a beacon beckoning man back to the primal world of organisms in an environment of birth, growth, physiological process and death. The tension between them which, according to Freud, sustains civilization, is very great and it is no wonder that many are unable to bear it and have 'nervous breakdowns'. In theory, at least, the regular practice of nudism should help, as the authority quoted above maintains, to restore some of man's lost integrity.

But there is another, and perhaps even more important, dimension to the virtue claimed for nudism. It is a rather nebulous one, although in some form or another it crops up in the writing of all enthusiasts, and is probably dependent upon experiencing nudism for full substantiation. The following passage by an American wife and mother who first dubiously tried nudism and later became a supporter, goes some way towards expressing it:

> You go home rejuvenated not only in body and mind. You get the feeling as you stand by your car and disrobe that with your clothes you strip off the ugly, dirty world and here alone is peace and brotherhood with your fellow man. Here you find friendly, cordial people, broad of mind, tolerant, respectful of persons. And when you do finally reach the understanding of the philosophy of nudism, you find your horizons unlimited, a great peace of mind, a richness in your enjoyment of life. You have found that freedom. And you bless the day you agreed to go to the nudist camp.

The chief idea expressed in this, and cognate pronouncements, is one of release. Removing your clothes symbolizes 'taking off' civilization and its cares. The nudist is stripped not only of garments but of the need to 'dress a part', of form and display, of ceremony and all the constraints of a complex etiquette. Strangely enough, he, or she, is also liberated from the rituals of sex. Flirtation, coquetry, calculation as to intentions, considerations of 'how far to go', of alluring or repelling posture, of 'what it will lead to' are all alien to the theory, at least, of nudism. Further than this, the nudist symbolically takes off a great burden of responsibility. By taking off his clothes, he takes off the pressing issues of his day. For the time being, he is no longer committed to causes, opposed to this or that trend, in short a citizen. He becomes, or seems to become, a free being once more, like a hind in the forest or a bird. It is this aspect of nudism which had made ritual nakedness symbolic of innocence to sects such as the Adamites.

It may be as well to say at this point that the experiences of the lady quoted above as regards finding nudist colonies populated by 'friendly, cordial people, broad of mind, tolerant, respectful of persons' does not fully accord with the historical facts. Maurice Parmelee in *Nudism in*

Modern Life (1929) gives various examples of nudists who failed to conform to this ideal pattern. He refers, for example, in a footnote to the 'nationalistic, militaristic and racial misuse' of nudism. Elsewhere he talks disparagingly of 'aesthetic nudism' and instances clubs in the twenties which suspended 'corpulent' members and others which only allowed members who were attractive and well-proportioned. Finally, he admits that racism, even in England, was not unknown. He describes a nudist society in which:

> ... the notion is prevalent that the nordic blond type is much better adapted for gymnosophy than the Mediterranean brunette type. When the persons sharing this notion gained control, they promulgated an edict that representatives of the South European races would not be admitted to membership. It is almost superfluous to add that these race bigots are bitterly antisemitic and would under no circumstances admit a Jew.

Parmelee is saddened by the human frailties of his fellow nudists but not surprised by them. Elsewhere he remarks: 'While some gymnosophists are very unconventional, many are, apart from their divergence from custom with respect to dress, dominated by convention.'

What, you may be wondering, is gymnosophy? It is the same thing as nudism, or rather it is an alternative name for the same thing. A phenomenon worth looking at briefly is the fact that the deliberate practice of nakedness in a habitually-clothed society has never been able, even though its lifetime has been brief, to find a stable name. In the early days in Germany, it was called simply and sternly '*Nacktkultur*' (naked culture). This term was soon superseded by others such as *Freiekörperkultur*, *Lichtkultur*, *Lichtfreunde* (free-body culture, light culture, friend of the light) and so on. In France, in the early days, terms such as *amis de vivre* and *naturistes* (friends of life and naturists) were popular. Maurice Parmelee suggested the term 'gymnosophy' (roughly, naked knowledge) and indeed subtitled his book *The New Gymnosophy* (the old gymnosophy, incidentally, was a sect of Hindu ascetics known to the ancient Greeks). In England and America during the thirties the terms nudism and nudist became standard. But not for long. In the post-war years, there has been a gradual swing towards the, originally, French expression 'naturism', which is now generally used to describe the movement and its practitioners. When the name of a thing keeps changing, the thing itself is usually unstable. An analogy is the continually changing term for an American negro. The crudely-racist 'nigger' was supplanted, with the first wave of reformist opinion, by the euphemistic 'coloured man'. Increasing ethnic pride led to the rejection of this in favour of the straightforward 'negro'. When this became contaminated by continued racial prejudice, the defiant 'black' was announced and is, at the time of writing, still the accepted term. But the successive proclamations of new, assertive terms and their subsequent corruption and dismissal really reflected the fact that the reality behind them had remained unchanged or at least unvanquished. As long as racist discrimination continues in America, men with pigmented skins will seek to discard old terms, which have become infected with prejudice, and find brave beginnings in new ones.

Nudism or naturism probably does not keep changing its name to escape external persecution but because of a deep sense of unease within the movement. Strictly speaking there is no such thing as a nudist. Everyone is a nudist – under his clothes. Everyone is a part-time nudist, bathing, dressing or undressing, and often in bed. Everyone has a bare skin. What *is* naturism? The practice of *not wearing clothes*. But this is clearly a negative concept, and what 'naturists' want to proclaim is something positive. At the back of the shifting designations can be seen the audacious concept that nudists or naturists disparage themselves by needing a group name at all. It is really the others, the overwhelming majority, who *do* wear clothes who should have a cult name. They should be called 'garmentists' or something similar, but can more than 99% of the human race really be the slaves of a neurotic fad? It is hard to see a way out of this dilemma. If being naked is really natural then how on earth can it be an 'ism' which implies a sect or cult? At Cap d'Adge, where my wife and I spent a week, the neighbouring, and much larger, conventional holiday centre is referred to by the naturists, with slightly defensive contempt, as 'the textile area'.

Cap d'Agde, near Beziers in the South of France, is, at the time of writing, the largest and most opulent naturist establishment in the world. It can cater for several thousand visitors, making it more a naturist town than, as it is designated in the brochures, a village. The public facilities are approximately what one would expect for a small holiday resort. There are two shopping centres which contain every kind of food shop and, it may seem paradoxically, clothing shops (though rather oddly, when we were there, no chemists). There is quite an ambitious restaurant, three or four cafés, a gymnasium, two swimming pools and even a discotheque, proclaimed in brave, fractured English as a 'nigth-club'. The beach has ice-cream and coffee stalls spaced along it. It is a far cry from the clearing in the woods of twenties nudism.

All day, when it is high summer and the weather, as is normal, is inviting, a line of cars passes slowly through the mechanical barriers bringing thousands of day-visitors to join the residents. These are mostly family groups and, in principle, unaccompanied men are only allowed in if they are members of an 'authorized' naturist establishment. We approached about lunch-time on a hot day in the back of a taxi hired at Beziers. There is no doubt that one of the key moments of an introduction to naturism is one's first sight of unselfconscious naked people. Our taxi edged towards the barriers and suddenly we saw a couple emerging from a wooden structure that was clearly administrative. The man was totally naked and the woman was wearing a bikini-bottom. They walked away together at the same moment that a boy of about fourteen, completely naked and tanned deep brown, pedalled furiously past on a bicycle. After that, we saw individual, or little groups of naked people, moving mostly in the middle-distance since we were on the fringes of the place and stuck in a panting line of smelly vehicles. Soon we saw numerous people, walking and talking, examining a boat, eating ices, playing, in the case of children, just as all the people one had ever known had done but, unlike any people one had ever seen before in the ordinary activities of everyday life, all stark naked. And, of course, the force of the word 'stark' was brought home. A body in the life of most people is a body with more or less fabric adhering to it. Here were bodies without fabric, without fur or feathers, more naked than animals – in fact, stark naked. But certainly not particularly erotically arousing or shocking – just stark and strange.

The next key moment in an encounter with naturism is, naturally, taking off one's own clothes. As prospective adventurers into naturism, two people could hardly be more different than my wife and I. She is in her thirties, tall, slim, attractive and unscarred. On the other hand, I am in my fifties, decidedly stocky and with an abdomen scarred and battered by surgery. I was none too happy about exposing my disfigurements to the world, but had decided that they would provide a good barometer as to the claims of the naturists. If, with my disadvantages, I still lost all self-consciousness, then there must be something in those claims. Feeling a little strange, but no more so than my wife, as she admitted, I undressed and we followed our host out into the bright sunshine and along a concrete path towards the chief shopping centre.

A little later we were shuffling along among thousands of naked people. Everywhere we looked were little naturists and big naturists, fat and thin ones, young and old ones. Each glance disclosed more bottoms and breasts than either of us had seen in the whole of our former lives. Everywhere gleamed clumps of pubic hair, gold and russet, brown and black. Nude couples, hand in hand, skipped past us into the waves. Enormous ladies, buttocks opulent as sugar-loaves, plodded resolutely towards the ice-cream stands. It was indeed hard to remain self-conscious in that active host comprising every kind and condition of mankind. And yet, not quite impossible. Perhaps a week was not long enough for a conclusive experiment, but my wife and I agreed that we never felt completely natural in the natural state.

Surprisingly, though we fall as readily into opposite corners on almost every issue as two boxers in a ring, my wife and I agreed about most things at Cap d'Agde. We agreed that there are certain indisputable delights. These are naked swimming and sunbathing and naked children, whose exquisite brown bodies tumble and splash everywhere. We also agreed that the austere pronouncements of the early apologists for 'nudism' to the effect that all erotic interest soon evaporates are far from true. It never evaporated at all for us and at the end of the week my glance was still tugged towards the median region of people's bodies. Apart from instinctual imperatives, there was the question of sheer curiosity. We discovered that what are coyly called the private parts are actually exceeded in variety only by that most public of parts, the face. Genitals are highly individuated and retain their capacity to magnetize (as faces do!). I never got used to raising my head from the sand and finding that I was gazing straight up between the parted legs of a woman. And my wife admitted that when three or four bronzed young men marched past us, thoughts unassociated with the beneficial properties of sun and air tended to cross her mind. But we also agreed that, in the last resort, you judge naked people by the same criteria as clothed ones. Character survives insignia. Indeed, at social gatherings, I found it quite easy to forget that half or more of our fellow guests were stark naked.

Social gatherings? Yes, that was a bit of a surprise. In fact, the incidence of parties on the little terraces was so great that reaching the beach became a test of grit and determination. 'Won't you join us for a drink?' rang out on every side and sometimes, after striding forth boldly from our flat after lunch, we only finally lurched onto the sand in time for a quick dip before dinner.

At these social gatherings, the chief topic of conversation was usually naturism. Naturists seem obsessed with their pursuit to an extent that renders their claim that it is 'simple and natural' seem suspect. Amazonian Indians don't spend their time at feasts discussing their naked condition. Among naturists there seemed to be an element of extreme self-consciousness, albeit cerebral, and of obsessive concern with their own practice and its implications.

'I think there are voyeurs about', was a typical remark, which might extract from a worldly naturist the laughing confirmation, 'Of course there are voyeurs about – I'm a voyeur myself!'

It slowly became clear, both from our own reactions and from inadvertent or even deliberate admission by 'old hands' that, far from being anaphrodisiac, as the founding fathers maintained and a few apologists still insist, naturism is suffused in gentle eroticism. Does this ever lead to sexual excess? We attended no orgies but there were hints that orgies occurred. As one man pointed out: 'After all, if you're naked, you're half way there already.' There were also postcard ads outside some of the shops in the shopping centres that, although discreetly worded, suggested quests for erotic adventure.

Undoubtedly relevant to the psychology of naturism is the answer to that question which occurs to everyone when 'nudist camps' are mentioned and which some people are still too shy to ask: don't the men have permanent erections? Oddly enough, the men never seemed to get erections at all. I didn't, and the whole time we were there we saw only one man with what might have been an erection although it might also have been simply a singular genital formation. Why don't male naturists respond in what might a priori be regarded as a natural way, to being surrounded by naked women, many of them attractive?

Probably the answer is that naturism, at least as practised at Cap d'Agde, does not represent a different way of life from that normally led by its practitioners but essentially the same way of life with the absence of clothes. Therefore the conventions governing everyday life persist and are simply modified, usually in the direction of greater control, to accommodate the changed conditions. Ordinary sexual response is not given freer expression but is subjected to unspoken rules even more firmly than it is in clothed society. Paradoxically, the 'sex-in-the-head' which so disgusted D.H.

Lawrence achieves its greatest dominance in a naturist establishment. Thus even fleeting physical contact is, in the ordinary course of daily life, avoided. This, in a crowded supermarket, for example, with people stooping everywhere to pluck tins from low shelves, takes a bit of doing. A speeded-up film of naturists doing their shopping would reveal a series of deft, if unconscious, avoidance manoeuvres. In our whole week there, I never so much as brushed against another person. All this exquisite weaving may be necessary to prevent the perpetual outbreak of overt physical eroticism, but it can hardly be considered natural. It follows then that this particular naturist establishment, at least, did not represent a society of naked people but of clothed people temporarily attired in nakedness. My wife and I found it exceedingly pleasant, and would be happy to spend more time at Cap d'Agde or a similar place again, but we agreed that it gets no closer to the innocence of Eden, or of the Amazon basin, than Times Square does.

In the twenties, Maurice Parmelee had great hopes for 'gymnosophy'. He conceived of a 'gymnosophic society' as a reformed society based on ideals of simplicity. Food and clothing would be rationalized and simplified. Architecture would be functional. Gardening and farming would be staple pursuits (although industry, a little hard to imagine in the naked state, also had a place). Entertainment and diversion would be of the do-it-yourself, folk variety. Morality would be high and human relations, in a society purged of visual insignia, would be far more democratic.

The actual historical development of the movement seems to have been rather different. Significantly, at Cap d'Agde my wife and I did not feel, and no one else expressed, that sense of 'release' which formed so conspicuous a part of the claims made by early naturists. This is undoubtedly because a place like Cap d'Agde, far from providing a radically different kind of environment (which can be supplied even by a humble clearing in the woods), really attempts to duplicate the amenities and essential characteristics of the greater society. It is not, in the Parmelee sense, a 'gymnosophist society' but a section of the greater society where people do not wear clothes. In spite of the contempt expressed by the naturists of Cap d'Agde for the neighbouring 'textile area', there seemed little essential difference between the two. Undoubtedly, the 'naturist village', because it was simpler and laid more stress on physical activity, was more agreeable than the 'stage-set' artificial fishing-village with its yacht marina and endless cafés and shopping parades where the bikini-clad holiday-makers shuffled about all day. But the difference was almost purely stylistic and not psychological. The naturists too had cars, dined in restaurants, sipped cocktails in cafés, danced in their own discotheques and lived much as urban man does everywhere today. There was no sense of forming an idealistic society apart. It was true that when, as occasionally happened, people from the 'textile area' found their way to the naturist beach and participated in the outdoor activities while stubbornly clinging to their bathing costumes, the absurdity of 'getting dressed' to go swimming was sharply emphasized. But, apart from functional messages of this kind, it was hard to see what Cap d'Agde really contributed to the problems of a civilization that has largely lost touch with its physical base.

Put in metaphysical terms, it can be said that naturism represents a revolutionary solution to the problem of body-alienation and that, like all revolutionary solutions, it contains the seeds of reaction. Largely by means of the device of adopting concealing clothing, the human race has devoted tens of millennia to harnessing its sexual energy for the task of constructing an elaborate technological culture. This historical movement cannot be undone, even if it were desirable to undo it, simply by spending a holiday in the nude once a year. True change in any sphere of human activity can only be evolutionary, can only be achieved by incorporating new principles slowly into the psychology and sociology of mankind.

So a trip to a naturist establishment is not a trip back in time to a lost, natural world, but simply a shift into a slightly different mode of civilized life. It does not take one back to Eden so much as into the ambience of a burlesque show. This seems to be even more the case in those American swingers' hotels where people meet for promiscuous sexual activity. So far from being reunited with their bodies and their instincts, they are merely arbitrarily abrogating, for a brief period, the rules and norms which still reign in their consciousness and their everyday lives. They are separating desire from emotion, thereby making their physical freedom more, not less, artifical.

All of which is not to say that there is no place for naturism. Its thoughtful, and indeed idealistic (with no senses of puritanism intended) practice probably has a part to play in the important quest for the reintegration of the genitals, and of instinctual life, into the human body. But it is probably a relatively small one. If Eden is a good place to be, it must be sought in the future, not in the past. We cannot return to it any more than we can return to any other period of history that nostalgia endows with almost certainly spurious charms.

EPILOGUE

Eden symbolizes unselfconscious existence and hence the animal world. Animals feel no shame. They do not have bodies. They *are* bodies. Any act of those bodies is an unambivalent expression of the nature of the animal. There is no moral discrimination. In a sense the animal has no independent existence. It does not distinguish between itself and the rest of the universe. It does not distinguish between itself now and itself then or in the future. Man lives. An animal *is* life. There are huge benefits to the animal stage. Since the animal does not inhabit time, it cannot know death in the way we know it. Since it has no means of discriminating between states of existence it may feel pain but it cannot undergo the kind of mental suffering we experience. Since it makes no moral judgements, it can enjoy untrammelled instinctual gratification. There are also great penalties. The animal is deprived of emotions which are dependent on a sense of continuity. It is barred from a sense of achievement. And it cannot, the greatest penalty of all, identify with processes that extend beyond its experience. Because it cannot objectify, it cannot survey. Although heir to all the delights of Eden, the animal is a prisoner in Eden. Only man, beyond the walls, is free.

Of course, the animal world is stratified and the consciousness of an anthropoid ape is clearly considerably more highly developed and subtler than that of a lizard. An amoeba and a dolphin are further apart than a dolphin and a man. It is quite possible, indeed, that dolphins and other aquatic mammals are potentially capable of the same kind of self-consciousness as man and may at some future time join us outside Eden. Then again, very primitive human communities, such as the

Tasaday, might be considered to share many qualities with the animal world although speech, which all humans have, is a crucial barrier. Broadly speaking, however, we can consider non-human life as unselfconscious.

Our clothes can be considered the walls of the Garden of Eden, remembering that, paradoxically, we are *outside* the walls when *inside* our clothes. Unhappily, however, we cannot return to Eden by the simple expedient of removing our clothes.

Clothes, in psychological terms, symbolize instinctual repression. Sexuality has provided the power to generate our cultural and scientific progress. But once instinct has been diverted from its primary tasks then it no longer has a definite goal. Thus shame engenders ambiguity. From ambiguity derives morality. And morality generates casuistry and conflicting aims and goals. An animal questions nothing. A human being questions everything.

Since shame is the progenitor of the cultural development that separates man from animals it is not surprising that the chief question, and hence moral dispute, that has always preoccupied man concerns sexual morality. Man differs from the animals chiefly in conscious regulation of his own sexuality. Undoubtedly, a powerful element in man's repudiation of, or at least ambivalent attitude towards, his own erotic drive stems from his wish to distinguish himself from the rest of creation. We are not brutes. We feel shame. Ergo, we are human.

But we have carried this key distinction to absurd and dangerous lengths. We have divorced ourselves from our instincts so conclusively that we are now menaced by their perverted expression. The blocked erotic instinct turns into destructiveness and, in our age, many thinkers have perceived that some of the most ghastly manifestations of human culture are fuelled by recycled eroticism. Channelled into pure cerebration, the sexual instinct may generate nightmares impossible in the animal world. Animals are casually cruel and are usually, not always, indifferent to the pain of other animals. Animals kill for food or, rarely, for sport but they do not torture, gloat over pain or exterminate. We do. What's more, we can tolerate our own ferocity.

What we cannot tolerate is our own sexuality.

Those who advocate censorship usually proclaim the need to suppress or regulate expressions of sex or violence. In a sense, these two manifestations represent opposites. Sex is, in its essence, the act of procreation or generating new life. Violence, in its cardinal manifestation, is murder or the termination of life. Those who object to violence may, of course, object to distressing or lurid depictions of natural as well as human violence. In rough schematization, however, we can say that birth and death are the subjects which aspirant censors consider unfit for human inspection.

There are two interesting considerations to be derived from this analysis. First, sex is pleasurable, physically harmless in all but its most bizarre manifestations, and its end product is renewed life, the next generation. Violence is painful or fatal, ugly, frightening and terminates or mars human life. It is odd that they should be bracketed together as unmentionable, and unrepresentable, things.

But it is even odder that the censors hardly ever succeed in banning violence and they almost always succeed in banning sex. Indeed, it is difficult to escape the feeling that they are not nearly as concerned about violence as they are about sex and that they often append the second term only to defend themselves from the charge of being motivated by simple prudery. In any event, the most cursory glance at our culture reveals that violence in all its forms is rampant in every branch of the media. Murder, war, torture, guns, swords, planes, tanks, bombs, fires, fists annihilate and mutilate legions daily on screens, stages and in the pages of books. Prim old ladies devour gory thrillers on the patios of hotels. Newsreels and television sometimes catch actual moments of death and torture, occasionally relaying them as they happen. There are, from time to time, murmurs of protest but in general it is accepted that wallowing in violence is compatible with our morality.

The situation with sex is quite different. We are widely supposed to have experienced a new liberation and acceptance of erotic physical reality since the last war. It is certainly true that books and films, and other media too, now discuss and represent things that would have been unthinkable only a few decades ago. National television, in England, from time to time projects fleeting images of naked people. In print, it is now the case that virtually anything can be said. But sex still lags a long way behind violence in either its appearance in art and the media or its tolerance by the public mind. In city centres, for example, it is common to see posters representing violence but never sex. It is quite acceptable to exhibit a twenty-foot tall representation of a soldier stabbing a bayonet through a woman. It would be considered utterly unacceptable to show the same couple copulating. The fact that representation and discussion of erotic matters is still far from free can be gauged by the enormous pornography industry. As with any black market commodity there is a black market in sex only because the free market does not supply enough to meet the demand. If there were not still a huge residual appetite for erotic accounts and representations, there would be no pornographers. There is, for example, no black market in violence. The appetite is adequately met by the respectable, free market and no one accuses the publishers of thrillers, say, of battening on filth. Why can we live with our own violence but not with our own sexuality?

The obvious answer is the one that has already been expressed in this epilogue and developed elsewhere in this book: man needs to harness erotic energy for civilization-building. Free-flowing sexuality must, therefore, be modified or even suppressed. This was Freud's view. But Freud also said that he stood for greater sexual freedom. In other words, the sexual repression = cultural development equation is no longer an unconscious one. It can, and to some extent it has been, critically scrutinized. But despite a wide-ranging debate in the twentieth century, and some relaxation of sexual taboo and censorship, our culture remains one in which unimpeded instinctual expression is outlawed. The representation and practice of sex arouses much greater horror than the representation and even the practice of violence.

What are the roots of this curious discrimination in favour of death rather than life? We are now far removed from animals. We no longer need to convert instinct into culture and we realize that truth. But a sense of the need to suppress free-flowing sexuality is still almost universal. Can it be explained as a cultural imperative? There are really only two satisfactory hypotheses to account for the sinister inequity between our response to violence and to sex.

The first is that human beings really hate and fear life and hence abominate the sexuality which propagates and extends it. This is not so far-fetched as it may, at first glance, seem, since such an attitude is a component of all world religions and actually constitutes the essence of some. If the universe is conceived as a struggle between debased matter and redeemed spirit, then flesh, as a part of matter, must also be debased and hence life is a pollutant. From this point of view, man's chief goal must be to escape life. This is not just a matter of dying since, to the Buddhist for example, life is very tenacious and if it is freed from its imprisonment in one material prison or body it will dive into another. This doctrine of reincarnation symbolizes the reality that the individual perishes in order to confer greater vitality on the species. As Schopenhauer pointed out, the ancient Brahmanical saying: 'Woe,

woe, the lingam (penis) is in the yoni (vagina)' laments the fact that when the act of generation occurs spirit is returned to its material prison. Can this be the feeling behind the repudiation of eroticism in Western civilization? It may well play a part but it is almost certainly a relatively small one. After all, for every death-oriented religious proposition, there is an equivalent life-asserting one, and for every pessimist artist or philosopher there are many life-affirming ones. The fundamental bias of our species, like that of every species, is to relish life and seek for more, not less, of it. What then is the second hypothesis?

It is that sexual energy is needed by the authorities of the world to maintain order. If we accept this proposition, then it immediately becomes obvious why the true obscenity of killing and violence has always been of less concern to those in power than the pseudo-obscenity of erotic acts. Death provides no scope for a network of regulations by which society can be manipulated. All the authorities can do about the dead is decree that they should be buried. But sex is a permanent fountain of dynamic energy, which can be tapped for social purposes by regulations concerning marriage, divorce, adultery, fornication, incest, homosexuality, bestiality, chastity, promiscuity, decency and so on. All those who wield power intuitively perceive that in the last resort their authority derives from the repression, and regulation, of sexuality, and that free-flowing sexuality is the biological equivalent of anarchy. All transferrals of power, all revolutions, are invariably accompanied by transformations of the regulations governing sexuality. And these are never, or never for long, in the direction of relaxation. Pre-revolutionary fervour and idealism may include 'free love' as one of its aspirations but with the reality of power comes the inevitable perception that truly free love would be incompatible with the maintenance of authority. Power may, of course, be used well or badly, and anarchy, in our present stage of development, might well be disastrous, but all administration is purchased with instinctual sexual energy.

We cannot return to Eden, to unselfconscious participation in nature and unimpeded instinctual gratification. This is another way of saying we cannot become animals again. Even if we go naked, we wear the 'mental clothes' of language and cultural inheritance. Is there anything we can do to mitigate the undoubted over-repression that characterizes Western, which really now means World, society? There have been a number of attempts in our century, and especially since the last war, to find radical solutions. The naturist movement has been discussed in this book. The American 'hippy' movement at its best represented a generous and lofty aspiration towards the recovery of spiritual values and erotic sanity. At its worst, of course, it perverted these goals ruthlessly. More recently, sex cults and groups have flourished and continue to do so. Contact magazines procure introductions between strangers for erotic encounters. Purpose-built clubs and hotels serve as arenas for orgiastic sex. Erotic entertainments proliferate. There has been, in the last decade, considerably greater social tolerance of 'irregular' sexual contact, that is casual sexual relationships, homosexual pairing and sex between the unmarried. But it is doubtful if any of these phenomena, or all of them combined, represent anything like a change of consciousness. They are more like safety-valves that permit the release of the erotic pressure that tends to build up to danger levels in well-fed and increasingly leisured societies. But safety-valves keep a system intact. They do not change it. And the need for change is urgent. We are menaced by new weaponry of unprecedented destructive power, enough, some people think, to annihilate all human and perhaps all other life on the planet. Our future will depend to some extent on whether we can achieve enlightened change in our attitudes towards, and hence relationship with, our own bodies and our own sexuality.

BIBLIOGRAPHY

Ballou, Robert O., ed., *The Bible of the World* (London, 1939; New York, 1973)

Beaglehole, J.C., *The Journals of Captain Cook* (London 1969; Stanford, 1974)

Berger, John, *Ways of Seeing* (New York, 1973; Harmondsworth, 1977)

Boccaccio, Giovanni, *The Decameron* (Harmondsworth, 1972)

Boileau, Jacques, *A Just and Reasonable Reprehension of Naked Breasts and Shoulders by a Grave and Learned Papist, Jacques Boileau* (London, 1678)

Brown, Normon O., *Life Against Death* (Middletown, 1959)

Chitty, Susan, *The Beast and the Monk* (London, 1974)

Clark, Kenneth, *The Nude* (Harmondsworth, 1970)

Danielsson, Bengt, *Love in the South Seas* (London, 1956)

Elkin, A.P., *Social Anthropology in Melanesia* (Westport, 1976)

Ellis, Havelock, *The Psychology of Sex* (London, 1933; New York, 1978)

Fisher, Seymour, *Body Consciousness* (London 1973; New York, 1974)

Flügel, J.C., *The Psychology of Clothes* (London, 1930; New York, 1976)

Freud, Sigmund, *The Complete Psychological Works of Sigmund Freud* (London, 1951; New York, 1964)

Gibbon, Edward, *Decline and Fall of the Roman Empire* (London, 1960)

Goodall, Jane, *In the Shadow of Man* (London, 1974)

Gosse, Edmund, *Father and Son* (New York, 1963; London, 1970)

Greenway, John, *Down Among the Wild Men* (London, 1974)

Greer, Germaine, *The Female Eunuch* (St. Albans, 1971; New York, 1972)

Kilvert, Francis, *Kilvert's Diary* (London, 1938–40)

Kira, Alexander, *The Bathroom* (Harmondsworth, 1976)

Kohler, Wolfgang, *The Mentality of Apes* (London, 1925)

Langdon-Davies, John, *The Future of Nakedness* (n.p., 1929)

Langer, Lawrence, *The Importance of Wearing Clothes* (London, 1960)

Longford, Lord, *Pornography: The Longford Report* (London, 1972)

Macdermot, Brian Hugh, *Cult of the Sacred Spear: Visit to the Tribesmen of the Southern Sudan* (London, 1972)

McLuhan, Marshall, *Guttenburg Galaxy* (London, 1962; New York, 1969)

Mead, Margaret, *Growing Up in New Guinea* (London 1931; West Caldwell, N.J., 1976)

Melville, Herman, *Typee* (Harmondsworth, 1972)

Morris, Desmond, *The Naked Ape* (London, 1967; New York, 1968)

Murphy, Yolande and Robert, *Women of the Forest* (New York, 1974)

Naipaul, V.S., *India: A Wounded Civilisation* (London, 1977)

Norwood, Clarence, *Nudism in England* (London, 1933)

Parmelee, Maurice, *Nudity in Modern Life* (London, 1933)

Rawson, Philip, *Erotic Art of the East* (Berkeley, 1977)

Rudofsky, Bernard, *The Unfashionable Human Body* (St. Albans, 1971; Garden City, New York, 1974)

Scott, G.R., *The Common Sense of Nudism* (n.d., 1934); *The Story of Baths and Bathing* (n.d., 1939)

Scutt, Ronald and C.L. Gotch, *Skin Deep* (London, 1974)

Senancour, *De l'Amour considéré dans les lois réelles et dans les formes sociales de l'union des deux sexes* (Paris, 1805)

Shuttle, Penelope and Peter Redgrove, *The Wise Wound* (London, 1978)

Stubbes, Philip, *The Anatomie of Abuses* (1583; Norwood, N.J., 1972)

Swift, Jonathan, *Gulliver's Travels* (London, 1974); *Poetical Works* (Oxford, 1967)

Walter, *My Secret Life* (New York, 1966)

Waugh, Evelyn, *The Loved One* (Harmondsworth, 1970)

Webb, Peter, *The Erotic Arts* (London, 1975; Boston, 1976)

Witkowski, G.J. and L. Nass, *Le Nue au théâtre depuis l'Antiquité jusqu'à nos jours* (Paris, 1909)

Wolfe, Tom, *The Kandy Kolored Tangerine Flake Streamline Baby*

Wright, Lawrence, *Clean and Decent* (London, 1960)

Yeats, W.B., *Collected Poems* (London, 1956)

Zuckerman, Sir Solly, *From Apes to Warlords* (London, 1978)

INDEX

ACKNOWLEDGEMENTS

The illustrations in this book were kindly provided by the following sources and are listed in the order in which they appear.

Between pages 32 and 33: Camera Press; Kunsthistorisches Museum, Vienna; Kobal Collection; Alan Hutchison Library; Alan Hutchison Library; Alan Hutchison Library; John Topham; Keystone Press; Popperfoto; John Topham; Rex Features; John Goldblatt; Rex Features; Cambridge University Museum of Archaeology and Anthropology; Australian News and Information Bureau; Popperfoto; Popperfoto; Camera Press; Chris Lund; Museum of Modern Art, New York; John Topham; British Museum; London; Rex Features.

Between pages 80 and 81: Rex Features; British Museum; Bridgeman Art Library; British Museum; British Museum; Rex Features; Kunsthalle Bremen; Frans Halsmuseum, Haarlem; Bridgeman Art Library; John Topham; Mander and Mitchenson; Rex Features; Rex Features; John Topham; John Topham; John Topham; Fox Photos; Mary Evans Picture Library; British Museum; Rex Features; Camera Press; Sunbathing Annual, 1955; John Topham; Rex Features; Pirelli; John Topham; Claire Leimbach.